The Science of Health & Healing

Also by Trevor Gunn:

'A Mother's Vaccine Dilemma
How to Make your Choice with Confidence'
ISBN: 978-0-9928522-1-4
www.vaccine-side-effects.com

'Vaccines – This Book Could Remove your Fear of
Childhood Illness'
ISBN: 978-0-9928522-1-4
www.vaccine-side-effects.com

Trevor Gunn BSc Hons LCH ACHom
Medical Biochemist, Registered and Practising Homeopath
www.achomeopaths.org

Currently Practising At:
The Dyke Road Natural Health Clinic, Brighton, UK
www.dykeroadclinic.co.uk
And
The Japan Royal Academy of Homeopathy, London, UK
www.rah-uk.com

Trevor Gunn BSc Hons LCH ACHom
Can be available for talks & presentations
Please contact:
enquiries@trevorgunn.com
Trevor has presented in the UK, Ireland, Japan, Egypt,
Lebanon, Iceland, and Croatia, and on National TV & Radio

The Science of Health and Healing

Trevor Gunn BSC Hons LCH ACHom

Published by

bolistic
promotions

Holistic Promotions

ISBN: 978-0-9928522-0-7

Published & Designed by:

Holistic Promotions
202 Carterhatch Road
Enfield
Middlesex
EN3 5LZ
United Kingdom
email@holisticpromotions.co.uk
www.holisticpromotions.co.uk

Distributor:

Lightning Source UK Ltd
Chapter House, Pitfield
Kiln Farm
Milton Keynes
MK 3LW
United Kingdom
Fax: 0845 121 4594
www.lightningsource.com

Acknowledgements

I gratefully acknowledge the support and patience from all of my dear family members, Jodie, Mirelle, Leon, Ylana and Tarnae in assisting the creative environment for me to work, to James Gunn and Agnes Gunn for all of their devoted parental support that makes life possible. I should also like to thank Phil Akilade, Colin Grant and Jamie Taylor in the arduous task of editing and encouraging my volumes of writing. Last but not least I extend my humble gratitude to all patients, students and participants of my lectures; they have equally given as much as I have received from the many experts I have encountered.

The Science of Health & Healing

"The body has a wisdom of its own, which is very much deeper than the mind. The mind is a late arrival. It does not know much yet. All the basic things the body still keeps in its control. Only useless things have been given to the mind..."

Osho

INTRODUCTION

There are 36,600 GPs in the UK, while in 1998 the first ever survey for the government shows that specialists in complementary and alternative medicine outnumber GP's with around 40,000 practitioners.

Peter Hain, The Secretary of State for Wales; 19 October 2004:

> "When our first baby, Sam, was born with eczema, various creams were prescribed. But they didn't work. Nor, when he developed asthma as well, did the prescribed steroid spray. It was only when - in desperation - we turned to homeopathy and radical changes in diet that both ailments went away."

An interesting anecdote, however, not by any means an isolated example; it is a fact that many people have succeeded in treating ailments with complementary and alternative medicine (CAM) when orthodox medicine has failed, and the popularity of CAM is steadily rising, its use doubling from 1994 to 2000. Data obtained from the Health Survey for England 2005 shows that 1 in 4 people had used CAM in the last 12 months and almost half the population of the UK had used CAM at some time in their life.

K.J. Hunt et al. 11/04/2010
International Journal of Clinical Practice. 64(11):1496-1502

An important question emerges: What is it that therapists of complementary and alternative medicine understand about the human body that either orthodox medical practitioners do not understand or are ignoring...and why?

There will of course be pros and cons to both holistic and orthodox medicine, and it is true that orthodox medical practice has its success, and pharmaceutical drugs have their use. But just as it would appear prudent for regulatory bodies, sitting within the apparently safe haven of modern medicine, to assess the limitations of holistic medicine, are we similarly aware of the limitations of orthodoxy, the consequences of its over-use and the extent of its potential dangers?

Studies reported in the Journal of the American Medical Association (2000) gave estimates of deaths in the USA caused by conventional treatments and drugs: They total 225,000 deaths a year from iatrogenic causes (from medical intervention), constituting the **third leading cause of death** in the USA, after deaths from heart disease and cancer, and way ahead of the next leading cause of death, cerebrovascular disease (strokes). The largest category by far, is non-error, adverse effects of conventional medications, 106,000; that is, **deaths caused by drugs** that were **correctly prescribed** for the condition that they were designed to treat.

More recent reports in 2009, by including studies in hospital settings, nursing homes, looking at the over prescription of drugs, surgical and drug errors, do in fact make modern medicine the **leading cause of death** in the USA.

'Death by Medicine'
Gary Null PhD, ND; Martin Feldman MD;
Debora Rasio MD; Dorothy Smith PhD, Carolyn Dean

Fine-tuning or transformation?

From the public portrayal of modern medicine one would assume that our medical advances have been extraordinarily triumphant at combating disease and all that is left, is to encroach into the exceptional instances of rare disease with equal therapeutic success.

The views of Antonio Coutinho, Director of Immunology Research at institutes in France and Portugal, suggest otherwise:

> "...centuries after Jenner's 'vaccination' and more than 100 years after Louis Pasteur's principle of 'attenuated' vaccines, we are still totally devoid of vaccines against chronic infections and against a large number of acute infections... **Obviously, the lack of clinical success means that our <u>understanding</u> of the immune system, despite decades of intense research, <u>still remains elusive...</u>"**

The rates of; cancer, autoimmune disease, allergies, and autism are on the increase, and in parts of the Western, world life expectancy is expected to decrease in the current generation. Are there fundamental principles of health and illness that have yet to be incorporated into the orthodox model?

Many of us have already experienced the benefit of a different approach to health care in the many forms of complementary and alternative medicine (CAM) and some may be able to understand the holistic rationale; the most pertinent questions may therefore be not whether their use is right or wrong, but compared to a pharmaceutical intervention, in which situations are they appropriate and in which situations are they not? It is of course possible that CAM is far more appropriate than many would dare to imagine and this necessarily leads us to a different understanding of health and disease.

The terms 'complementary, alternative or holistic medicine' do however refer to a plethora of preventative and therapeutic interventions, involving therapies, supplements, diets, exercise and life style, they incorporate a multitude of diverse approaches. However there are some fundamental principles common to many, in particular the understanding that

> *...the body possesses highly evolved mechanisms designed to heal and keep you alive,*

...a seemingly incontrovertible facet of human life, yet, it is an aspect that is almost completely disregarded by the pharmaceutical approach to the treatment of illness.

The body is of course highly intelligent and is designed to continually maintain optimum health; even symptoms of disease are beneficial examples of the drive towards health.

Indeed many avenues of scientific research into the human physiology increasingly concur with the foundations of holistic medicine illustrating the intelligence of the body in health __and__ disease. As such, the understanding of the mechanisms behind the intelligence of the body in disease gives a significant biological basis to most of these alternative therapies. Understanding, the intelligence of the human body in disease, enables a completely different interpretation of the biological mechanisms of illness than our current orthodox pathology (study of illness) allows and as such provides a more congruent basis for understanding illness from the perspective of the holistic therapist.

The dominant medical paradigm views most illnesses and therefore symptoms of illness as being malfunctional artefacts requiring the intervention of drugs, to try and stop these symptoms, i.e. these abnormal functions. If in fact the body has an ability to maintain health and to self-heal, then our concepts of how and why the body functions in disease need to be radically reframed. Such a perspective, by incorporating biological detail and overview, gives intelligent meaning to the process of disease and enables the integration of holism and biology.

For patients and therapists, both orthodox and alternative, the goal is simple and remains the same for everyone; optimal health for ourselves and loved ones, now and into our, hopefully, long-lived future, the question of course is, how do we achieve that? Can we prevent disease and successfully treat illness with current pharmaceutical drugs or are there fundamentally safer and more effective ways of using billions of years of evolved human physiology with holistic medicine and is it possible to have an effective mix of the two?

The public, however, in searching for answers find themselves in a sea of contradictory information, between an increasingly popular holistic health movement and an equally persuasive, yet apparently opposing, technological orthodoxy. For many years these disciplines have been evolving along very different paths; a holistic, wherein the body is viewed as an integrated mind, body and spirit, requiring therapists that are able to work with the intelligence and interconnectedness of our systems. In apparent contrast we have the modern biochemical world of cells, genes and microbes providing the scientific basis of real illnesses, dividing the body into parts requiring specialists and serious pharmaceutical drugs that are able to put a mal-functioning body right.

For years these worlds have existed independently as though concerned with distinctly separate phenomena, yet they offer descriptions of the same world, the world of health and illness.

Apparent discord between orthodox and so-called alternative medicine often develops from interpretations arising from a difference in context, each having a different perspective of the facts. This book looks at the human body through the eyes of a modern day biochemist and a holistic therapist, and by looking at certain examples shows how these two apparently opposing world views can be integrated to give a coherent picture of physiological intelligence.

With the biological detail from modern science as well as the overview obtained from holistic medicine this book goes on to clarify the principles of holistic medicine in a manner that is accessible to most of us with a cultural background in modern medicine. By integrating knowledge of orthodox science and holism, we are demonstrably more able to choose effective strategies for healing disease, improving our health and thereby safely and effectively avoiding future illnesses.

CHAPTER ONE

1 Moving to a new more effective health paradigm requires us to clarify the existing paradigm that is almost part of our cultural DNA

"The processes of disease aim not at the destruction of life, but the saving of it."

Frederick Treves, 1905

Many aspects of modern science are beginning to unite, elucidating a picture of living processes that are also more congruent with the principles of holistic health. Philosophies once considered poles apart are finding themselves converging; it is from the apparently divergent disciplines of biomedical science and holistic medicine that we shall build our picture of health and disease.

How can we transform our thinking about Health and what are the limitations with our current thinking about Health?

In order to delineate this more encompassing health paradigm we have first to recognise that there already exists, across all spectrums of society, from medical professionals to the lay public, accepted concepts of disease and immunity. These concepts have become so pervasive and subtly dominant in our culture that they are now firmly seated in our consciousness, influencing much of our thoughts, fears and desires.

Currently, we may no longer be aware of our own medical opinions; rather than see medical perspectives as evolving concepts, they have become fundamental truths of the nature of life. Unless we have had an extensive and alternative medical training, then most of us will have become the 'non-expert' experts of orthodox medicine.

Throughout this book we shall be distinguishing our new paradigm from the current orthodoxy by looking at three fundamental issues:

- ➢ Symptoms of disease & immunity
- ➢ Germs the infectious agents and causes of disease…and
- ➢ Genes, the determinants of our function and ultimately our mal-function.

1.1 An Orthodox Perspective

A fundamental concept inherent within the system of orthodox medicine is the perception of most symptoms of illness as malfunctions of the body.

Human beings are seen as sophisticated machines and from time to time things will go wrong, and when they do, we produce symptoms of illness. Just as a machine that starts to malfunction will need the expert engineer to fix it, our symptoms of illness show us that we need fixing by the doctor, it is necessary for us to be put right. Like a household appliance that no longer works, a leaking pump, a blown fuse, a broken belt, the only way we can function normally again, is if it we are fixed and if not, things can only get worse.

In such human instances of malfunction, we are also likely to deteriorate and therefore in the case of an illness, this can ultimately lead to our death. Therefore medical expertise will also involve sophisticated means of screening for early signs of malfunction, with the development of diagnostic technology able to detect increasingly smaller deviations from the norm. Then with the use of pharmaceutical drug intervention the ability to put things right before they deteriorate further. Best of all, medical experts will aim to develop preventatives such as vaccines, able to put things right, almost imperceptibly, before anything even starts to go wrong.

1.2 Intelligent by design - the intelligence of the body in sickness

However, orthodox scientists know that ordinarily the human body responds intelligently to changes in the external environment in ways that allow the internal cellular surroundings to remain fairly constant, this is of course vital, because the functioning of the body can only occur within a certain range of internal conditions.

All forms of life from single celled algae to mammals have mechanisms that are capable of responding to changes in temperature, humidity, levels of nutrients, oxygen, carbon dioxide, acidity, light, perceived danger etc and of course none more so than the sophisticated physiology of the human being. So if, for example, the external environment gets colder, our internal system heats up to compensate, if we have insufficient intake of water then the systems retain more water, etc. This process of internal balancing is called homeostasis and in fact, the body can only remain alive whilst these coordinated responses are working.

However, as soon as these reactions become uncomfortable they are classified as symptoms of illness, in looking at symptoms in more detail it is apparent that most of these responses are no less intelligent than the ongoing homeostatic mechanisms of the body in health, symptoms are in fact examples of the body's drive towards optimum health.

We shall be looking in detail at this issue throughout this book, demonstrating that symptoms of illness are not examples of physiological malfunction but are precise coordinated reactions occurring when the body is stressed beyond its normal limits. Each of those symptoms has a specific function in helping the body to adapt and respond to its environment. In fact the presence of symptoms indicates that the body is already engaged in adaptation and repair. The body may be going through a necessary process of learning in its adaptation to a new environment, or responding to harmful elements that need to be avoided.

By looking at the overview of a disease process, as is more common in holistic therapy (holism; the whole picture) one can make observations with regard to what causes a symptom reaction, how are the various parts of the body integrated in their responses, how is one system assisting the other systems, and additionally observe the outcome of these reactions, i.e. what is the body trying to achieve in its response. With such an overview it is possible to gain some understanding as to the purpose of symptoms in their drive to maintain health and their attempts to adapt to adverse circumstances. Most holistic therapies are based on this wider perspective and consequently utilise techniques that are able to work with these reactions as opposed to simply trying to stop them.

This approach places almost all holistic therapies together and distinctly apart from orthodox drug therapy; hence they are often grouped together under the banner of alternative medicine, even though they are in fact many and varied. The underlying philosophies frequently appear to be shrouded in esoteric language not easily accessible to the orthodox mind; however understanding the body's ability to self-heal is a fundamental principle they all have in common.

Pharmaceutical drugs or any medication designed to stop symptoms will ultimately stop the self-healing process itself. As the body attempts to respond again, this prompts the prescription of further medication, which could ultimately lead to drug dependency or worse still, deeper health problems.

To understand symptoms of illness scientists need to take an overview of what causes symptoms, what the symptoms are responding to, what is the goal of the symptom and how that integrates with other systems of the body. In other words in order to understand health and illness, scientists need to take a more holistic view as well as their own detailed research of cell biochemistry. Healing would involve both helping the response of the body and ascertaining what the body is responding to so that the causes can be eliminated or reduced.

This would appear to be a somewhat unorthodox view rarely utilised in conventional medicine, however, it is a point of view already adopted by many traditional researchers. Conventional scientists are in fact looking at symptoms as a positive response to trauma, responses that have evolved over millennia; therefore the question emerges, as stated in The New Scientists Oct 23, 1993...

> *"Should we treat the symptoms of disease, or are they an aid to recovery?"*

...The article goes on to comment on research being carried out by other scientists, claiming that ...

> *"The underlying message is uncontroversial enough: human beings and their illnesses are the products of a long evolutionary history. Yet modern medicine, for all its high-technology treatments and preventive strategies, has so far largely ignored this fact."*

Randolph M Nesse (Medical Doctor and Professor at University of Michigan Medical School) and George C Williams (Professor Emeritus University of New York, Member of US National Academy of Science) have written the book 'Evolution and Healing'. In referring to the symptoms of the body as 'evolved adaptations' they and others have coined the term 'Darwinian Medicine'.

The book charts the many examples of how the human physiology responds to environmental trauma and how the symptoms have evolved for the benefit of the patient.

For example, the benefits of diarrhoea in the evacuation of intestinal pathogens, how the vomiting in morning sickness can protect the developing foetus from toxins and the physiological response to a sprained joint, they ask:

> ➤ Are the symptoms an incidental consequence of the trauma, or an adaptation to promote healing?
> ➤ How is the sensation of pain produced? ...And what is its role in the healing process?
> ➤ Therefore <u>what harmful consequences may result from stopping the symptoms?</u>

They go on to state...

"Only by answering these questions can we choose the correct treatment."

Pharmaceutical intervention for the most part aims at halting the symptom responses of the body in illness, this may be applicable when the body is no longer capable of compensating BUT the orthodox practitioner is now faced with the question of deciding when it is appropriate to stop symptoms and when it is not, because symptom suppression is potentially dangerous to the patient, giving that symptoms are highly evolved mechanisms designed to keep you alive. Additionally practitioners would be obliged to research therapeutic interventions that can enhance the symptom response, thereby speeding up the healing process, as well as only focussing on medication that can suppress responses. Ultimately medical researchers are compelled to search for the true causes of illness which are often environmental and lifestyle.

Therefore this is not a question of deciding whether we are advocates of holistic medicine or of orthodoxy, but a need to discern when the suppressive approach of orthodox medicine is useful and when is it not.

Similarly, holistic therapists are responsible for having the ability to discern when to refer patients for orthodoxy, i.e. when the symptom responses of their patients are no longer compensatory. Of equal importance, the holistic practitioner would be greatly helped if they understood the detailed biology underlying the intelligent responses of the body in illness, which would therefore add to the scientific basis of their therapy.

The challenge of course is to understand the intelligence of the body in the many scenarios of illness that present in the real world, therefore further books will look more specifically at; autoimmune illness, cardiovascular illness, blood sugar balance, diabetes, obesity, cancer and mental health illness from the perspective of - the intelligence of the body in health **_and_** illness.

CHAPTER 1 - SUMMARY

> ➤ Modern medical concepts are culturally ingrained and have been adopted by most of the general public even, in the non-medically trained.

> ➤ Basic principles of medicine suggest that microbes (germs) cause disease, symptoms of illness are a sign of mal-function and the ultimate susceptibility to disease is genetic, over which you have no power.

> ➤ The holistic paradigm of the intelligence of the body in disease acknowledges that symptoms of disease are in fact attempts of the body at healing and re-balancing.

> ➤ The understanding of the human body in illness, (the study of pathology), would need to be re-framed to accommodate the fact that many symptoms are intelligent reactions produced when the body is stressed beyond its normal limits.

> ➤ With such a perspective therapists would be obliged to look at what the body is reacting to and therefore the causes of illness.

> ➤ Orthodox medicine as supported by a pharmaceutical approach to health care views the symptom as a mal-function and therefore needs to be stopped, consequently symptoms are suppressed.

> ➤ We therefore need to investigate what are the consequences of suppressing the highly evolved symptom reactions that occur during an illness, and if there a more effective approaches?

CHAPTER TWO

2 How the human body manages toxins

Looking at the body intelligence concept in a little more detail we shall consider the following example: Toxicity in human metabolism, our ability to eliminate toxins in health and illness, and consequently raising the question; do germs (e.g. bacteria, fungus, viruses etc) cause disease or does the toxic environment invite the germ.

2.1 Toxic waste - a fact of life

There are of course many external influences on the body that we have to adapt to, temperature, light, humidity, pollutants, etc; however, there are also those issues created by our own internal metabolism. 'Metabolism' being the word to describe the overall chemical reactions of the human body - taking in food substances to be oxidised (burnt) in the presence of oxygen, thereby releasing energy for our daily functions, and the incorporation of these food substances to renew and create the structures of the human body.

The accompanying accumulation of by-products is generally toxic and consequently these waste products need to be eliminated, the production of this waste, effectively toxins, occurs even if we could conceivably ingest no toxins at all, therefore toxin elimination is something the body is extremely efficient at doing... it has to be, in order to stay alive.

When dealing with health and illness the issue of toxicity within the body is paramount. A toxin is any substance that can adversely affect the function of your cells and there are many kinds of toxins affecting different cells in a variety of ways.

Therefore, because our normal metabolism produces toxins, we have many mechanisms in place to eliminate these potentially harmful substances out of the body and if these toxins are particularly dangerous they will have to go through a chemical process of deactivation and attachment to carriers, often in the liver, before they are eliminated from the body.

The following processes as well as performing other functions, also serve as the main mechanisms of elimination.

a. Perspiration - Skin
b. Respiration - Lungs
c. Urination - Kidneys
d. Defaecation - Bowels

2.1.1 Ingestion of toxins

As well as the normal production of toxins from our metabolism, we also know that toxins can be ingested into the body, for example: Through our digestive system from food and drink, there are food elements that are themselves toxic as well as pesticides and other chemicals in what we eat and drink; through our lungs via air pollution and smoking, and through our skin from cosmetics, pollutants in washing water and other elements in contact with the skin. All of which will need to be eliminated as described above.

2.2 Assembling the parts - an introduction to holism

"Science is built up of facts, as a house is built of stones; but an accumulation of facts is no more a science than a heap of stones is a house."

Henri Poincaré, Science and Hypothesis, 1905

For the purposes of toxicity and elimination, the body can be described as having an inside and outside. The inside, being separated from the outside, by a physical membrane, our 'skin'. Pierce the skin and you will expose our internal environment, blood, tissues etc to the external environment.

Our skin covers the entire body, and at the mouth, the skin continues into the cavity of the digestive system, via the lips, maintaining this barrier into our digestive tract. The skin lining the mouth is different from our external skin; in the mouth it is a mucous membrane, but nevertheless it is a skin continuous with your outer skin covering the body. This membrane continues through the length of our digestive tract through the throat, stomach, small intestine and large intestine until it reaches the anus, whereupon it forms a continuous membrane with our skin once again. It is as though the digestive tract from mouth to anus forms a continuous tube through the body, much like the whole though a doughnut.

It is important to have a general understanding of the inside and outside of the body from the perspective of your skin and mucous membrane. Although the body can be divided into parts, a whole body perspective of 'in and out' allows us to appreciate the purpose of various symptoms in disease and the priorities of the body in terms of physical development, protection and ultimately survival.

2.2.1 Diagrammatical representation:
Digestive tract running through the body

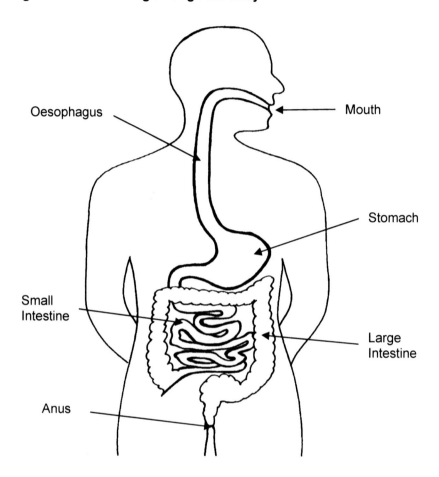

Anything within the cavity of our mouths can still be considered to be outside of our bodies, i.e. it is not until a substance passes across this membrane that it is actually internalised. Consequently anything in your stomach and intestines can be considered to be outside of your body until it passes across the membrane lining the stomach and intestine. If you were to swallow something relatively small and indigestible like a glass marble, this would pass right through your digestive tract: mouth, throat, stomach, small intestine and large intestine and be passed out through your anus and at no time would it have been internalised into your body.

This is the way we shall consider inside and outside of the body for the purposes of this part of our discussion. A similar situation can be said to exist for other parts of the body also, the lungs, ear, nose and throat also bladder and kidneys.

2.2.2 Diagrammatical representation
Respiratory tract and Urinary tract running into the body

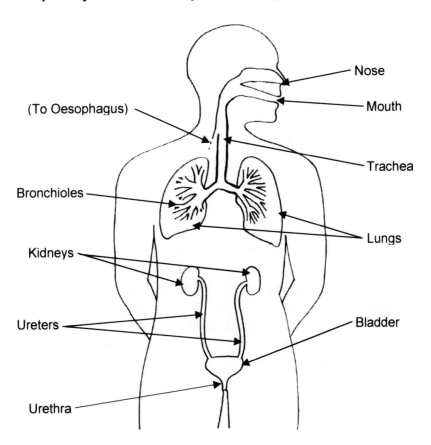

Now these structures do not have tubes that pass right through our bodies like the digestive system, but generally consist of tubes that are blocked off at their ends that also separate the internal tissues by a membrane that is once again continuous with the outer skin.

In the elimination of toxins, the waste products of our metabolism are usually eliminated into these spaces: The large intestine for defaecation, the kidneys and bladder for urination, the skin in perspiration and the lungs during respiration, whereupon they are then expelled completely from the body.

This toxin elimination is a very important part of our immune function and the presence of the **membrane** is an important structure involved in these processes. There are elements present on these membranes that are important for the functioning of the membrane: mucus and other secretions, acid or alkali solutions, enzymes, immune chemicals, non-specific antibodies (immunoglobulins), white blood cells, cilia (fine hairs), bacteria, fungus and viruses.

2.3 Symptoms - Function or Mal-Function?

"Disease is not a meaningless "error" of nature or biology but a special program created by nature over millions of years of evolution to allow organisms to override everyday functioning and to deal with particular emergency situations; they are wonderful programs and, if understood correctly, provide the individual and the group with a way to deal with "out of the ordinary circumstances".

Dr Ryke Geerd Hamer

We know that certain factors can lead to an accumulation of excess toxins in these external body spaces, digestive tract, upper ear, nose and throat, lungs, bladder, etc:

1. **Sudden or gradual increase of ingested toxins: -**
   From our diet, drug habits, environmental pollution etc.

2. **Reduced capacity of organs to eliminate: -**
   Due to physical or mental & emotional stress

3. **Nutritional deficiencies including water: -**
   Contribute to the inability of the body to carry out basic eliminatory functions.

4. **Direct suppression of our elimination responses: -**
   From the use of antiperspirants etc.

If we are able to eliminate these toxins as fast as they accumulate then our normal function of perspiration, respiration, urination and defaecation is sufficient to eliminate toxicity.

If however our normal functions were unable to eliminate toxins fast enough then the accumulation of toxins would provoke an increased elimination response from your body:

- Vomiting and diarrhoea.
- Respiratory mucus with coughing, sneezing and nasal discharge.
- Increased sweating and urination, with increased concentration and odour.

The function of these responses at this stage would be to increase toxin elimination as distinct from the normal physiological responses of perspiration, respiration, urination and defaecation: These increased responses are now associated with feelings of discomfort, we now experience **symptoms** of 'dis-ease'. There may be some debate as to when you decide some reactions are symptoms, for example profuse sweating in extreme heat or physical activity will not be considered a symptom of illness because the reaction is not disproportionate to the activity of the person. Diarrhoea, vomiting, coughing and sneezing will, more often than not, be considered symptomatic of illness unless there is an immediate and benign cause.

Generally before the onset of symptoms you would have been able to eliminate all toxins through your **normal 'function'**, and therefore with no discomfort (perspiration – skin, respiration – lungs, urination – kidneys, defaecation - bowels) but at this stage, because of an excessive build-up of toxicity, an increased response is necessary, therefore **'symptoms'** are experienced; sweating and urination with increased odour and concentration, vomiting, diarrhoea, respiratory mucus/cough/sneeze etc.

2.3.1 Microbes and their association with toxicity

With the increased toxins within these spaces of the body the altered toxic conditions now encourage other microbes to multiply which brings us once again to the question of the role of microbes in disease. These microbes proliferate as a result of the underlying condition and therefore not the primary cause, they may help to clean up the environment and return to normal conditions, but with their concomitant waste they may however also add something to the toxicity.

Although these microorganisms are present in the toxic environment they were not responsible for the toxicity in the first place, the causes of these particular illness symptoms were the factors that lead to the original accumulation of excess toxins in these external body spaces:

1. Sudden or gradual increase of ingested toxins: -
   From our diet, drug habits, environmental pollution etc.
2. Reduced capacity of organs to eliminate: -
   Due to physical, mental or emotional stress
3. Nutritional deficiencies: -
   Contribute to the inability of the body to carry out basic eliminatory functions.
4. Direct suppression of our elimination responses: -
   From the use of antiperspirants etc.

However from an orthodox perspective the focus is almost entirely on the identification of the microbe so that it can be killed. But because there will always be many microbes present at the site of the symptom response, it was however very difficult to decide what microbe was the actual 'cause' and so certain criteria are used to decide which microbe is associated to which disease and from this it is assumed to be the primary 'cause'. These criteria were developed in the late 19th century by the German scientist Robert Koch.

2.3.2 Koch's Postulates

In 1890 the German physician and bacteriologist Robert Koch set out his celebrated criteria for judging whether a given bacteria is the cause of a given disease. These criteria are taught to this day and are used by scientists to help them decide whether a given bacteria can be defined as being responsible for a particular disease. Koch's criteria brought some much-needed scientific clarity to what was then a very confused field.

Koch's postulates are as follows:

➢ The bacteria must be present in every case of the disease.
➢ The bacteria must be isolated from the host with the disease and grown in pure culture.

> ➢ The specific disease must be reproduced when a pure culture of the bacteria is inoculated into a healthy susceptible host.
> ➢ The bacteria must be recoverable from the experimentally infected host.

However, Koch's postulates have their limitations and so may not always be the last word. They may not hold if:

> ➢ The particular bacteria cannot be "grown in pure culture" in the laboratory.
> ➢ There is no animal 'model' of infection that accurately mimics the human illness in which to carry out experiments.
> ➢ The bacteria can only cause disease when introduced into the body in ways that do not naturally occur.

In addition a harmless bacterium may cause disease if:

> ➢ It gains access to deep tissues via trauma, bites, injections, surgery, etc.
> ➢ It is present in an immuno-compromised patient.

And even in bacteria that appear to be demonstrably pathogenic (associated with disease), in fact not all people infected by the bacteria develop disease, sub-clinical infection is usually **more common** than clinically obvious infection, i.e. although many individuals have the bacteria **most show no symptoms of disease**.

Similarly illnesses presenting with the same symptoms will often be associated with many different microbes or even none at all. For example influenza-like symptoms have been associated with flu viruses, respiratory synctial viruses, bacteria and most are not associated with microbes at all.

Despite such limitations, Koch's postulates are still used as a benchmark for deciding which type of microorganism is responsible for which disease. However, until further investigations are carried out, this will only tell us which microbes are present at the time of certain diseases but cannot tell us as yet whether they 'caused' the condition or whether they are the 'result' of the condition. For example we will always find flies around cow dung deposited in the grazing fields of cows, but flies are clearly not responsible for depositing them, flies are correlated to cow dung in cow fields though not causative, consequently they are part of the effect but not the cause.

However, much of our orthodox diagnoses and interpretations of the cause of infectious disease, do not account for the exceptions to the rule and the fact that the exceptions far outweigh the rule.

For example Hib, Meningococcal and E.Coli bacteria are all supposed to cause meningitis yet most of us have these bacteria within our systems all the time with no symptoms of illness. Evidence of viruses; HPV, HIV, herpes and polio though found in huge proportions of the population, yet again for the vast majority they are associated with no symptoms of disease.

We seem to be in need of a more accurate and up to date concept of disease, one that enables us to understand how microbes create no symptoms of disease in the vast majority yet appear to be associated with illness in a small percentage. It may be that much of our current concepts of infectious disease are actually stuck in the past.

CHAPTER 2 - SUMMARY

> ➢ Toxins accumulate in the body from the continual internal metabolism of the cells, in addition to toxins that invade from the outside.

> ➢ The body functions to eliminate these toxins every second of the day, through perspiration, respiration, urination and defecation.

> ➢ These eliminatory functions pass these toxins from inside the body across the membranes and skin to the outside.

> ➢ The outside of the body will include the digestive tract, lungs, urinary tract and skin.

> ➢ If toxins build up on these membranes, defined as outside the body, there will be an increased elimination effort resulting in symptoms of elimination; vomiting, diarrhoea, coughing, sneezing, etc.

> ➢ These symptoms are reactions to the problem of toxicity and not problems themselves.

> ➢ Microbes, bacteria, fungus and viruses can accumulate at these sites of toxicity and are not the primary cause of the symptom response.

CHAPTER THREE

3 Immunity and Infectious disease a historical perspective

Given the reality of our current understanding of the role of micro-organisms in the body, the general concept of infectious disease appears to be fundamentally outdated.

This historical context will create a wider perspective, illustrating how medical knowledge is developing and what aspects appear to be outdated.

3.1 How and when did we lose sight of what nature has been trying to tell us?

Both the general public and medical professionals are in general agreement about the mechanisms of infectious disease, including the basic principles of how to avoid and treat these illnesses. Most people believe that microbes, (bacteria, viruses, fungus etc.), invade us from the outside, thus causing the infectious illnesses; with some microbes being more virulent than others and consequently more dangerous than others.

We have also been led to believe that we are open to infection at any time and although we can do a certain amount to stay healthy, some microbes can affect and kill even healthy people.

Therefore we are told that the best way to avoid infectious illness is to actually develop immunity to that illness. It is thought that immunity can be obtained by two methods:

1. Naturally, by exposure to the microbe and therefore developing symptoms of the illness, the condition itself would provide life-long immunity.
2. Or acquired, artificial immunity, through the use of vaccines.

According to method one, for example contracting 'measles' naturally and developing symptoms of measles, including the development of the measles rash etc, this would confer life-long immunity to the measles microbe. By our method two, artificial immunity, the use of measles vaccine, such as with MMR, would hopefully create artificially acquired immunity to the measles microbe with little or no symptoms of illness.

It is generally believed that natural immunity carries a certain amount of unquantifiable risk; it is possible that you could suffer any one of the many serious 'side-effects' known as 'adverse effects' from the illness, but we could not say for sure which, if any, would happen to you.

Blindness, deafness, brain damage or even death could happen as a result of measles infection. Some infectious illnesses themselves for example paralytic poliomyelitis are far more serious than typical measles. It is therefore acknowledged, by many people within the orthodox medical community, that vaccine-induced immunity although not as effective is potentially safer than naturally acquired immunity.

But what is the evidence for these theories of immunity and disease, and from where do they come?

3.2 Germ theory - what 'lies' beneath - The historical and underlying concepts of infectious disease

3.2.1 Pasteur and Béchamp

A cursory glance at medical history will reveal the name of Louis Pasteur, born 1822 in Dole, France, his name forever immortalised on a day-to-day basis in 'pasteurised' milk – named in his honour. As described in most conventional medical history texts, he has been credited with having transformed medicine, his contributions being that:

> ➢ He showed that airborne microbes were the cause of disease.
> ➢ He built on the work of Edward Jenner and helped to develop more vaccines.

However, a closer look at historical records will reveal otherwise, the basis of germ theory with the discovery of microbes was in fact developed and originated by other scientists and their conclusions regarding the causes of illness were very different from that of Pasteur. Germ theory itself was postulated years before Pasteur had claimed it to be his own and so having copied the work of others Pasteur took several more wrong turns before developing theories of germs and infectious disease. Pasteur's theories were however more acceptable than competing theories in the 19th century, and certain elements of the general public, medical community and government, all had an agenda, they were looking for a hero to champion their cause and that hero was to be Louis Pasteur.

In the West, medical theory with regards to infectious illness was actually consolidated with the work of Antoine Béchamp when he took up the study of fermentation (1854). He was a contemporary of Pasteur and to place their beliefs in context we shall look at the perennial question asked by scientists and philosophers both then and now:

> ➢ What were the origins of the universe, life and effectively ourselves, how and when did it all begin?

At the time of Pasteur and Béchamp, approaches to this question could generally be divided into two:

> ➤ One theory was that the substance of the universe was at some time created out of nothing and that 'creation out of nothing' was either spontaneous or due to the work of some kind of omnipotent God and that this phenomena could happen at any time. It was used to explain the mechanism of some diseases and the appearance of simple life forms in decayed substances etc.

> ➤ The other perspective being, that life had evolved out of substance that was always present, an evolutionary point of view. That is to say, the stuff of the universe, the planet and life on earth had always existed in some way, shape or form and had slowly evolved into forms of ever increasing complexity to what we see of life today. Life was not and could not be created spontaneously out of nothing. This was often considered to be the more 'scientific' view.

In the 19th century at the time of Béchamp and Pasteur, the commonly held doctrine, was that of 'substance out of nothing' and was called "spontaneous generation", a view supported by many scientists including Pasteur.

However, Béchamp not content to ascribe certain life processes to the theory of spontaneous generation studied three biochemical phenomena:

1. Sepsis
2. Fermentation
3. Grape diseases.

He demonstrated that there were small organisms involved in all of these processes, organisms that he later called 'microzymas', (effectively what we now call microbes). These microbes actually lived within the material of the substances of the above examples, digesting nutrients and producing waste products, existing like tiny animals in an ecosystem of food, water, shelter and toxic waste. He also demonstrated how they could be transferred through the air to contaminate other samples. Although this had been suggested before, Béchamp was the first to demonstrate this through scientific experimentation.

At this point he had not distinguished the various forms of microbes from each other i.e. fungal cells, bacteria, viruses, etc, but was however the first recorded scientist to demonstrate the effects of microbes, showing how they were able to exist and therefore interact within the larger 'host' organism and how their by-products would have subsequent effects in their host.

In the examples given:

> **Sepsis** – when a wound becomes septic producing pus: Bacteria and white blood cells destroy and digest dead cells and foreign debris at the site of an injury and the waste products of this cellular digestion forms the green pus seen at the site of a septic wound.

> **Fermentation** – sugar solution into alcohol: The small organisms are yeast cells which would feed off sugar, and the waste product of this sugar digestion is alcohol, thereby it appeared that under certain conditions sugar solution would turn into alcohol. Whereas in fact alcohol is being produced by the digestion of sugar by yeast cells.

> **The grape disease** studied by Béchamp was caused by certain microbes on the skin of the grapes which digest the grape juice extract and excrete waste products that affect the health of the grapevine and more importantly the quality of wine produced.

In 1857 Béchamp had irrefutably demonstrated the activity of these microbes and the concept of this microbial activity was therefore used to explain the mechanisms of the above processes. This was 'the' giant step forward in our understanding of microbes in fermentation and microbial diseases. Prior to Béchamp, scientists including Pasteur, explained fermentation as a simple 'spontaneous' chemical transformation without involving living microbes.

The deficiency of Pasteur's knowledge as compared to Béchamp is also apparent when we consider other experiments of Béchamp. Béchamp was able to demonstrate the activity of microbes in mixtures that had previously no microbes present; Béchamp concluded that these microbes were able to enter via the passage of air. However other scientists including Pasteur said this was due to microbes 'spontaneously' emerging. Pasteur's theories and experiments are clearly documented to have been years behind Béchamp.

In fact in 1859, two years after Béchamp had conducted his experiments and one year after publishing the conclusions of those experiments, Pasteur was still referring to the activity of microbe fermentation as "taking birth spontaneously" and therefore not acknowledging the passage of microbes in the air. Pasteur lacked the conceptual framework of Béchamp that would give him the ability to design experiments that could demonstrate the activity of microbes, yet it was Pasteur that had laid claim to having first discovered and demonstrated the existence of microbes in the air.

Pasteur carried out very little original experimentation and has been widely acknowledged as having plagiarised the work of Béchamp. In the 1940's book by R.B. Pearson originally published under the title "Pasteur, Plagiarist, Imposter", Pearson describes a meeting of research scientists at the Sorbonne University in Paris, Nov 22, 1861. Here Pasteur had to admit to knowledge of Béchamp's work whilst previously claiming credit for the proof of microbe theories as his own.

RB Pearson, in "Pasteur, Plagiarist, Imposter".

Dr M.L. Leverson MD PhD MA an American Physician, discovered some of professor Béchamp's writings in New York and immediately realised they had been published before Pasteur. He travelled to France to meet Béchamp and in a lecture entitled Pasteur, the Plagiarist, 1911 outlined Béchamp's claim to priority and added the charge that Pasteur had deliberately faked an important paper.

He said in part:

"Pasteur's plagiarisms of the discoveries of Béchamp, and of Béchamp's collaborators, run through the whole of Pasteur's life and work…"
"Finding how readily the 'men of science' of his day accepted his fairy tales, published in the Annales de Chimie et de Physique 3rd S., Vol. LVIII, there is a section entitled Production of Yeast in a Medium Formed of Sugar, of a Salt of Ammonia and Phosphates.
The real, though not confessed, object of the paper was to cause it to be believed that he, and not Béchamp, was the first to produce a 'ferment' in a fermentative medium without albuminoid matter. Now mark, I pray you, what I say – the alleged experiment described in the memoir was a fake – purely and simply a fake. Yeast cannot be produced under the conditions of that section! If those of my hearers or any physician having some knowledge of physiological chemistry will take the pains to read this section of Pasteur's memoir with attention, he will see for himself that yeast cannot be so produced, and he can prove it by making the experiment as described."

"…I cannot but believe that the exposure I am making of Pasteur's ignorance and dishonesty will lead to a serious overhauling of all his work."

Dr Leverson goes on to say…

"From the outline I have now given you, you may form some idea of the ignorance of the man who, for more than thirty years, official medicine has been worshipping as a little god. But this is only a small part of the mischief perpetrated. Instead of making progress in therapeutics during the past thirty or forty years, medicine – outside surgery – has fearfully retrograded, and the medical profession today is, in my judgement, in a more degraded condition than ever before in it's history."

However even this admission in the company of other researchers that Béchamp had already proved the existence of microbes did not stop his continued self-proclaiming as the discoverer of the activity of microbes.

Paul de Kruif in 'Microbe Hunters' speaks admirably of Pasteur...

"Pasteur invented an experiment that was – so far as one can tell from careful search through records – really his own. It was a grand experiment, a semi-public experiment, an experiment that meant rushing across France in trains; it was a test in which he had to slither on glaciers"

An experiment carried out in **1864** as recorded in the 14th edition of the Encyclopaedia Britannica showing how **Pasteur proved the existence** of... "organisms (microbes) with which ordinary air was impregnated".

However, it was a phenomena **already proved by Béchamp, seven years earlier, in 1857.**

It was in fact from the ideas of Béchamp that eventually lead Pasteur in the 1870s to conclude that:

> ➢ Microbes would cause illness after having infected the person via their passage through the air.
> ➢ Each specific microbe would cause an illness that was unique to that microbe.

This was the "Germ Theory of Disease" discovered first... supposedly by Pasteur as claimed by ...Pasteur.

According to the principles of 'germ theory', diseases were caused by the entry of microbes into the body from an external source, and were therefore called 'infectious diseases', each specific microbe causing its own specific disease. Therefore if somebody has measles illness, a measles microbe from the environment must have infected him or her and this microbe could be the only cause of measles. Another individual with for example chickenpox would therefore have to have been infected by a separate chickenpox microbe and this microbe is only capable of producing chickenpox illness and not measles.

This germ theory of disease, as with the theory of the passage of microbes in the air was again something that Pasteur claimed to be his own, even though in fact "germ theory" had been suggested long before. A fairly comprehensive summary of germ theory was postulated by M.A. Plenciz in 1762, 100 years before Pasteur had popularised it as having been his own, Plenciz stated:

> *"There was a special organism by which each infectious disease was produced, that microbes were capable of reproduction outside of the body, and that they might be conveyed from place to place by air".*

More recently, in 1993, according to Gerald Geison of Princeton University, examination of Pasteur's laboratory notebooks reveals that there were astonishing discrepancies between his notes and published writings, Geison states…

> *"Pasteur lied about the numbers involved in trials and about the production of the anthrax vaccine later used in a public trial, all of which helped both him and later his Pasteur Institute in Paris to become extremely wealthy and famous".*

Sylvie Simon writes of the works of Dr Philippe Decourt, Ethyl Douglas Hume, G Gerald Geison, Xavier Raspail, Daniel Raichvarg and others; from probing many authenticated research papers they reveal that Pasteur claimed for himself discoveries made by others and with the help of accomplices he doctored unfavourable experimental results and tyrannically refused to discuss them.

> ➢ *The drama of a 12-year-old child who died as a consequence of the vaccination revealed the dishonesty of Pasteur and his*

colleagues. On 16 October the child died. An inquiry under Professor Brouardel sought the cause but the lofty, titled, professor was a friend of Pasteur. Brouardel, in agreement with Roux, decided to falsify the evidence before the inquiry. In Les Vérités Indésirables - Le Cas Pasteur, Philippe Decourt records that it was a matter of avoiding official acknowledgement of a failure that would entail, according to Brouardel, "an immediate step backwards in the progress of science" as well as dishonour to Pasteur.

➢ *Pasteur vigorously opposed Henry Toussaint's theories and practices, which he said were ineffective and dangerous. To prove that his vaccine was better he agreed a protocol of experiments that would come to fruition on 28 August 1881 at Pouilly-le-Fort, near Melun. On the appointed day Pasteur confided to his associates that he would not use his own vaccine but Toussaint's. Who today is aware that the Pouilly le Fort experiment was no more than a hoax?*

3.2.2 Germs, friend or foe?

In any event, plagiarism and historical inaccuracies aside, Pasteur had popularised the germ theory of disease and in so doing placed the responsibility of illness on the infecting microbe, the 'germ'. The germ was said to enter the body from an external source, causing illness in the unsuspecting individual and was therefore said to be the primary cause of infectious illness.

It is worth noting at this point that Pasteur had never managed to prove or demonstrate that these illnesses were actually caused by infecting microbes, i.e. microbes that were not already present within the system. The idea that illness was caused by a microbe infecting the human body from the external environment was just that …an 'idea'.

Pasteur's theories suggest that if you have a pathogenic microbe (a 'disease-causing' microbe) that you did not have before, then it must have come from the outside and because microbes do not change form, it could not have been produced from other microbes already within the person. This is known as 'monomorphism', one definitive unchanging physical form, for each type of microbe. Therefore, once within the body, these microbes are able to multiply and the fear is that they could equally be given to others, thus spreading disease.

Béchamp on the other hand, went on to show that the microbes responsible for the diseases that he observed were actually already present before the initiation of the disease, he therefore deduced that the most important factor was the nature of the host material, i.e. the constituents of the bodily fluids and tissues upon which the microbes grew and multiplied. According to Béchamp it is the medium in which the microbes live and feed that determine whether the microbe produced substances that would enhance the health of the individual or whether they produce toxins that would exacerbate symptoms of disease. He also demonstrated that health conferring or benign microbes could therefore change into pathogenic microbes according to the nature of the patient's cellular environment.

Indeed Béchamp, and other scientists that followed, concluded that the micro-organisms involved in disease processes were in fact cleaning up the internal environment; they do not live off healthy living tissue but only diseased and dead tissue.

The ability of microbes to change form is termed pleomorphism and was an inherent part of Béchamp's observations and teachings; this was to be confirmed later in the 20th century by other scientists; Dr Gunther Enderlein, Dr Rife, Dr Gaston Naessens and Dr Wilhelm Reich, with microscopic techniques able to view live tissue samples.

Most observations of cells are conducted with light microscopes, the samples are usually thinly sliced and/or stained so that the various components can be seen by passing light through them against the background, but this means that the samples have to be killed, preserved and fixed in a suitable material.

However scientists working with live blood samples, use what is called 'dark-field' or 'dark-phase' microscopy, a different lighting technique is employed where the samples are not stained or killed and they are able to observe microbes changing into these different forms according to the nature of their environment; the more acidic, the less oxygenated and the more polluted the bodily fluid, the more we find associated microbes. As acidity and toxicity levels increases and oxygen concentrations decrease these microbes grow larger and accumulate protein reserves as an adaptation to their environment and practitioners are able to remedy diseases by addressing the conditions that create internal toxicity.

Researchers today using dark field microscopy are able to diagnose illness by observing these changes in microbes that are normally resident in each person, and are able to remedy diseases by addressing the conditions that create these imbalances.

These facts have been largely ignored by the present orthodoxy, mainly because they appear to undermine their own perspective and approach to treating illness. Orthodox interpretations tend to think of microbes as static elements unable to change form, ' monomorphism', and that pathogenic microbes are either present or not and that healthy human blood is sterile and therefore free of microbes. Therefore, the way to address illnesses with the presence of microbes is simply to kill them.

However, modern microbiology has in fact refuted all of the original assumptions of the monomorphic tradition, even though those doctrines still dominate our clinical medicine. In orthodox medical texts pleomorphic organisms are now acknowledged to exist, for example the rickettsia organisms involved in typhus. In addition, as published in the Journal of Clinical Microbiology, August 16 2002, conventional microbiological methods, have demonstrated the existence of populations of pleomorphic bacteria in healthy human blood.

Even from orthodox interpretations of illness, there are also known disease phenomena that would suggest a soil theory takes precedence. The theory of a 'carrier of disease' makes an allowance for the fact that all individuals carry potentially disease-causing microbes and yet do not have symptoms of illness but are in fact perfectly healthy; polio viruses, haemophilus influenza bacteria, meningococcal bacteria are associated with life threatening conditions, many are present within all of us yet we experience no symptoms of disease.

It is also known that a carrier can subsequently become ill from the previously present, though apparently dormant, microbe, in spite of which the medical establishment rarely questions the nature of this change. If carriers can subsequently become unwell from resident microbes, then a medical approach to treatment must involve an understanding of how that person became susceptible to the germ, it is therefore likely that killing the germ would leave the susceptibility unaltered.

For example in Australia with modern disease notification records and where families are more apt to live in isolation on their vast farmlands, children have been documented as having contracted chickenpox and other childhood illnesses when there has been no contact with anybody for months yet alone with anyone with chickenpox that could have 'given' them the illness. The standard incubation periods, in which the microbe can be harboured within an individual before symptoms are manifest, are usually estimated at around two to four weeks maximum. It is clear that these microbes exist within us for much longer periods and therefore the onset of symptoms may not be caused by the infecting microbe, but by a change in the internal environment of the patient. Once these changes have occurred the patient becomes susceptible to illness and opportunistic microbes proliferate.

In the NHS Public Health Network newsletter, 16th May 2002 Birmingham UK, under the heading 'Predisposing factors' there were concerns as to the reported cases of measles, none of the normal factors that could have caused the outbreak appeared to exist. The report stated that:

> ➢ None of the reported cases of measles were immunosuppressed i.e. none were taking immune suppressive medication.
> ➢ None had a history of overseas travel.
> ➢ None had a case of measles in their family or had contact with a known case.

This highlights the possibility that some individuals may develop measles from within; not necessarily caught from external sources. Almost 150 years after the soil theory of Béchamp, reports of pathogenic microbes that exist within the body become news worthy.

3.2.3 Seeing things differently to see different things

Therefore even though there appears to be only a subtle difference, the concept of disease according to Béchamp takes on a radically different flavour to that of Pasteur's germ theory. As far as Béchamp is concerned, microbes are present all the time, they are in and around us, and it seems there needs to be a significant change to the substances in which they grow, in order for them to multiply and therefore become associated with symptoms of disease. Diet, toxins, hormones, acidity, emotions, hydration, etc all influence the environment in which microbes live and grow in the human body and this environment, we shall call the 'soil' of the microbe. Like the soil of farmland, the nature of the earth and the climate around the earth, this determines what can be grown there.

From this perspective the substances in which the microbes grow, the "soil", takes on the greater significance, and not the presence or absence of these microbes, this we shall therefore refer to as Béchamp's "soil theory" of disease.

Béchamp's 'soil theory' relies upon the understanding that:

> ➢ There are changes in the proportions of existing microbes that can be associated with symptoms of disease, for example

small numbers of fungal cells are tolerated within the body but if you kill off large numbers of bacteria, with for example antibiotics, a greater proportion of fungal cells will dominate and create illnesses associated with fungus.

➢ Microbes can change from one related type to another - from health conferring microbes to microbes associated with disease. This change in type is what is known as 'pleomorphism'.

➢ In addition, there are also bacteria that produce certain healthy substances in certain circumstances but produce toxins if forced to live in other conditions for example in oxygen depleted environments.

If, as according to Béchamp, microbes do behave in this way, then of course illness cannot be avoided simply by avoiding contact with microbes in the external environment, even though they can be transferred from one person to another, they can equally be produced within. Similarly, killing microbes associated with disease without addressing the conditions that are creating them will not stop more of them from being produced from the many millions of microbes already within the body.

3.2.4 Florence Nightingale

A very interesting counter-argument to germ theory comes from an unlikely source, Florence Nightingale (1820-1910), 'the lady with the lamp'. Famous for her contribution to nursing during the Crimean war, she gained many insights into the nature of disease. Medical history tells of a rather subsidiary role for nurses, although highly commendable, nursing has nevertheless been portrayed as rather secondary to the function of 'real doctors'. Florence Nightingale was however more outspoken than we have been generally led to believe. The voice of Pasteur may have been immortalised and Florence Nightingale relatively obscured, however, it appears as though she had some strong opinions regarding the theories of infectious disease.

Florence Nightingale did in fact endorse a perspective of infectious illness akin to that of Béchamp and published a counter-argument to the germ theory, in favour of a "soil theory" of disease. She acknowledges the influence of the human condition on the microbes, where microbes change from one type to another and therefore potentially pathogenic microbes are always present within an individual. Published over **17 years before Pasteur's claim to have originated the germ theory of disease**, further evidence that 'germ theory' was in fact common knowledge within the medical fraternity long before Pasteur had claimed to originate the idea himself.

Florence Nightingale…

"Is it not living in a continual mistake to look upon disease as we do now, as separate entities which must exist, like cats and dogs, instead of looking upon them as the reactions of kindly nature against the conditions against which we have placed ourselves?

I was brought up by scientific men to believe that smallpox was a thing of which there was once a specimen in the world, which went on propagating itself in a perpetual chain of descent, just as much as there was a first dog or pair of dogs, and that smallpox would not begin itself anymore than a new dog would begin without there having been a parent dog.

Since then I have seen with my eyes and smelt with my nose smallpox growing up in first specimens, either in closed rooms or overcrowded wards where it could not by any possibility have been "caught" but must have begun. Nay, more, I have seen diseases begin, grow and pass into one another. Now dogs do not pass into cats. I have seen for instance, with a little overcrowding, continued fever grow up, and with a little more, typhoid fever, and with little more, typhus, and all in the same ward or hut.

For diseases, as all experience shows, are adjectives not noun substances. The specific disease doctrine is the grand refuge of weak, uncultured, unstable minds, such as now rule in the medical profession. There are no specific diseases, there are only specific disease conditions."

Using the analogy of cats and dogs Florence Nightingale states that if illnesses are defined by microbes and these microbes are monomorphic, i.e. could not change from one type to another, then they could not begin out of nothing and one could not be created from the other, a cat could not be created from a dog and neither of them could be created without a parent cat or dog. However her experience shows that illnesses do behave like this, illnesses appear to start and change from one type to another simply by changing the conditions of the patient.

Illnesses, according to Florence Nightingale, are approximate descriptions of the nature of the patient and how they react to the conditions in which they live. She categorically states that an illness is therefore not a 'thing', what she calls a noun substance and cannot be defined by the nature of an unchanging infecting microbe, but disease is determined by the nature of the patient and their diseased conditions. A doctrine that was however viewed as erroneous by the medical establishment and even today according to the Florence Nightingale Museum Trust, London, they quote:

> *"Like her friend, the public health reformer Edwin Chadwick, Florence Nightingale believed that infection arose spontaneously in dirty and poorly ventilated places. This mistaken belief nevertheless led to improvements in hygiene and healthier living and working environments."*

It is of course interesting, that her 'mistaken belief' led to improved health.

Historical anecdote paints a rather interesting picture of the ultimate beliefs of Pasteur, Lionel Dole (1965) in his writings on the history of vaccination:

"Most people cherish their delusions even more than their other ailments. As Thomas Edison was fond of saying: 'There is no expedient to which Man will not resort to avoid the hard work of thinking.'

The germ theory and the idea that 'germs can be conquered by vaccines', was one of the most greedily grasped of all such expedients. It was so much more modern and scientific than the fuddy-duddy idea of mending our ways or atoning for past errors. Man wants to believe that the maladies he brings upon himself are all due to those terrible germs, which, being unable to sue for libel, are the ideal scapegoats. What a tremendous debt we owe to Louis Pasteur, the Microbe Man!

And yet Pasteur himself, at the end of his life, was quoted by his old friend, Prof. Renon, who attended him in his final illness, as having said:

"Bernard was right. The germ is nothing. The soil is everything."

It cannot be believed that this final scientific utterance of Pasteur's is not authentic, but it is not inscribed on the wall of his tomb, nor have we ever heard it quoted on the radio."

However, Béchamp's theories have since been relegated to obscurity, often described as "the lost chapter of biology" and concomitantly the theories of Pasteur have dominated, until perhaps, a more recent resurrection.

3.2.5 Why germ theory and why Pasteur?

"I have had my results for a long time: but I do not yet know how I am to arrive at them."

Karl Friedrich Gauss

Quite why Pasteur's views dominated so strongly has been fertile ground for many a conspiracy theory, however, an already susceptible population with given fears, desires and a mechanistic world view were in need of such a rationale to support their existing state of mind. This was the time of the industrial revolution, machines were what we understood, and phenomena in the natural world were going to be far easier to explain by making comparisons to our newfound technologies.

During the time of Pasteur a mechanical world developed rapidly, with applications in almost every sphere of life, transport, consumer goods, farming, communication etc. People were beginning to explain their world by using machine-like analogies; the body itself was nothing more than a sophisticated machine. Blood transported by a pump - the heart, through the tubes and valves of the blood vessels, muscles acting on levers, nerve impulses acting like electric currents through the wiring of our nerves. We were a long way from understanding the interconnectedness of our systems and the effects of our emotions and mental faculties on the body. And as promoted by Descartes since the 17th century, consciousness itself was nothing more than a ghost within the mechanical body and for some people nothing more than an effect of the mechanical body itself.

By the time of Pasteur in the 1870's, all Western Europe was more or less industrialized, the coming of electricity and cheap steel after 1850 further speeded the process. According to Professor G Rempel of Western New England College, The Industrial Revolution may be defined as the application of power-driven machinery to manufacturing.

Between 1780 and 1860 many textile processes were mechanized. By 1812 the cost of making cotton yarn had dropped nine-tenths, and by 1800 the number of workers needed to turn wool into yarn had been reduced by four-fifths. And by 1840 the labour cost of making the best woollen cloth had fallen by at least half.

The steam engine provided a landmark in the industrial development of Europe. The first modern steam engine was built by an engineer Thomas Newcomen, in 1705, to improve the pumping equipment used to eliminate seepage in tin and copper mines. In 1763 James watt, an instrument-maker for Glasgow University, began to make improvements on Newcomen's engine. In 1774 the industrialist Michael Boulton took Watt into partnership, and their firm produced nearly five hundred engines before Watt's patent expired in 1800. Waterpower continued in use, but the factory was now liberated from the streamside where water mills had previously been the source of factory power.

The power of the steam engines were then harnessed in the development of steam trains and the coming of the railroads greatly facilitated the industrialization of Europe. After 1800 flat tracks were in use outside London, Sheffield, and Munich. With the expansion of commerce, facilities for the movement of goods from the factory to the ports or cities came into pressing demand. By 1830 a railway was opened from Liverpool to Manchester; and on this line George Stephenson's "Rocket" pulled a train of cars at fourteen miles an hour.

As early as 1831 Michael Faraday demonstrated how electricity could be mechanically produced, however through the nineteenth century the use of electric power was limited but the electrification of Europe proceeded apace in the twentieth century.

The ideas linking the function of microbes within the human body to nutrition, toxins, hormones and emotions were slightly more sophisticated than popular 19th century Western thinking. In many ways these notions sit far more comfortably within the realms of present day holistic thinking and the interconnected universe of modern physics. They were however too advanced for the machine-like analogies used to explain the workings of the human body in the 19th century. Béchamp was going to find it hard to translate his ideas to the man on the street; this may have contributed to the popularity of Pasteur's germ theory and the relative demise of Béchamp's soil theory.

However, there may be other considerations regarding human behaviour that would account for the popularity of Pasteur. There is, within us all, a powerful resistance to change, an inertia and momentum that makes it easier to keep on doing what we've been doing. This particular human phenomenon would seriously influence our choices, given the following options:

> A 'germ theory' approach would place the responsibility for the illness on an external agent of disease; the solution would lie in the extermination of the microbe, with no requirement to change anything on our part. Germ theory would give us the option to take no responsibility for our situation in our treatment of disease.

> Adopting a 'soil theory' of disease (where microbes create symptoms of disease according to the conditions within the body) would lead us to acknowledge the role of diet, nutrition, hormones, toxins, lifestyle, etc. As such, addressing the problem of disease would require change on our part.

For many individuals in both 19th century Europe and equally in today's society, we have to consider what would be the most attractive option, would it be the one that allows us to blame something else and take no responsibility for our state of 'disease'? As such, the disease would have nothing to do with 'us'; we could combat the disease by simply annihilating the germ. Consequently we could make disease a thing that exists outside of us, the result of something that had nothing to do with us, therefore requiring remedial action that did not involve 'us' having to do anything as drastic as 'change'. It was not through scientific enquiry, research and experimentation that lead us to embrace Pasteur and marginalize Béchamp, therefore… was it a result of this psychological desire for Pasteur to be right?

If, as promoted by Pasteur, infecting germs were primarily responsible for illness then the way to treat the illness would be to eradicate the germs (kill them by the use of toxic chemical agents) and avoid infection by avoiding contamination i.e. by avoiding contact with people that are infected. The disease becomes the microbe; they become synonymous with each other, to have measles is to have measles virus and to have the virus is to have the illness. Even though most people have viruses and bacteria and do not have the disease, because having the virus and to having the illness are in fact two separate issues. We can therefore talk about the possibility of giving someone the illness because in the Pasteur paradigm, the illness is no longer anything to do with our susceptibility or state of health, but some 'thing' that we can catch and transfer from one unsuspecting host to another.

We can be given an illness like an inanimate object, an item of clothing or a piece of machinery, equally the illness itself becomes externalised as some 'thing', no doubt, that if malfunctioning, could be left on the physician's desk to study and investigate. 'It' can be sorted out whilst the patient is able to deal with more important things and no doubt carry on doing the same things that created the illness in the first place, so that with the right drug the illness will be fixed. As such 'it' will have nothing to do with their life; undoubtedly somebody else would have given 'it' to them. This may seem the more attractive option, rather than blaming oneself, far easier to blame someone else, some irresponsible or unsuspecting individual responsible for spreading disease around the community.

If on the other hand, as demonstrated by Béchamp, the soil, i.e. our susceptibility, (the state of health of the individual) is primarily important for the contraction of an infectious disease, then treatment relies upon restoring balance and addressing the primary cause of this susceptibility. This would involve addressing issues of nutrition, sanitation (i.e. reduction of toxicity), mental and emotional wellbeing, physical rest, relaxation and other environmental factors. Therefore, according to the principles of Béchamp, you could never in fact contract anything that you were not already susceptible to and you could never resolve an illness simply by killing microbes. The illness would be inextricably linked to you.

At this point in history in the late 19th century there were no mass produced vaccinations, no antibiotics, no large pharmaceutical companies and therefore, on the face of it, no real scope for commercial conspiracy over and above the opposing commercial interests of the orthodox medical profession and the natural health, hygiene and food industries; yet, as a culture we invested in one approach far more than in the other. The approach was obviously that of Pasteur's.

Did we invest in this approach because of the available evidence of what actually worked or was it a calculated investment in an approach that if successful would reap many within the profession financial benefit and the governing authorities, power to deal with illness by simply handing out medication? Germ theory was not only an attractive option for individuals but also for governments, the 'success to effort' ratio appeared infinitely greater in the Pasteur paradigm than in Béchamp's.

In the Pasteur paradigm, where germs infect people and cause disease, governments were faced with the possibility of dealing with society's ills by simply investing in the production of the correct medication for the correct disease. This could then of course be administered en masse for a relatively small investment per individual; we would have the prospect of immediate reductions in disease, within the term of government.

Government would have the possibility of success, without the tedium of having to deal with all those inconvenient, social and environmental issues of sanitation, food, shelter and social well-being. A germ theory of disease made the solutions to our troubles seem so much easier, and during the industrial revolution of 19th century Europe there were many social problems.

"They ruined us...They conquered continents.

We filled their uniforms... We cruised the seas.

We worked their mines...and made their histories.

You work, we rule, they said...We worked; they ruled.

They fooled the tenements...All men were fooled."

Douglas Dunn

The Industrial Revolution brought with it an increase in population and a shift from country to town dwelling. Between 1800 and 1950 most large European cities exhibited spectacular growth. At the beginning of the nineteenth century there were scarcely two dozen cities in Europe with a population of 100,000, but by 1900 there were more than 150 cities of this size.

The rapid growth of the cities brought some apparent advantages to the population but not without considerable cost to most people. The factory towns of England tended to become rookeries of jerry-built tenements, while the mining towns became long monotonous rows of company-built cottages, furnishing minimal shelter and little more.

The bad living conditions in the towns can be traced to lack of good brick, the absence of building codes, and the lack of machinery for public sanitation. But, it must be added, they were mainly due to the factory owners' tendency to regard labourers as commodities and not as a group of human beings.

Generally speaking, wages were low and hours were long, whilst working conditions were unpleasant and dangerous, with many businesses exploiting child-labour. For many, illnesses were a direct result of their living conditions; however, the wealthy factory owners owed their wealth to the exploitation of this new social class, their workers. Government usually favoured the factory owners; therefore reform and protective legislation was a long time coming and only after considerable public pressure in the form of coordinated unions and new socialist political opposition.

Eventually public health measures were developed, but in the 19th century the <u>medical</u> paradigm adopted by the government, was one wherein illnesses were caused by attacking microbes...

...governments were prepared to search for the magic bullet, but less prepared to improve the social conditions that directly lead to illness, especially if ultimately that was to be at the expense of their wealthy friends.

Commercial interests in the 19th century played a huge role in promoting the germ paradigm, and still do, with the concomitant search for commercially successful drugs in an attempt at the eradication of disease.

However, if Béchamp were correct, then diseases in our communities could only be dealt with by addressing those environmental issues: Workers hours would need to be cut, minimum ages introduced, pay increased, housing and sanitation improved, nutritious foods made readily available, and worse still, given the individual nature of susceptibility, therapeutic intervention would have to be tailor-made to each individual. All of which entailed far too much work and far too much investment from the government's affluent supporters for the uncertain prospect of their workers future health.

"I do not know of any environmental group in any country that does not view its government as an adversary"

GH Brundtland 1989
Three term Prime Minister of Norway (1981, 1986, 1990)
International leader in sustainable development & public health.
Served as the Director General of the World Health Organization

We as individuals wanted germ theory to be right, as governments and commercial business owners, we needed it to be right, we had our agenda... and our hero, Pasteur, was more than willing to champion the cause. An expert in self-publicity and adept at promoting what we wanted to hear, Pasteur, was clearly not the first to develop these ideas, nor the most knowledgeable; he was, however endorsing the right ideas, in the right places, at the right time, and more than willing to make financial profit from the whole endeavour.

"Let me tell you the secret that has led me to my goal. My strength lies solely in my tenacity"

Louis Pasteur

In March 1886 after enquiries into many deaths from his rabies vaccine Pasteur told Dr Navarre:

"From now on I won't accept discussion of my theories and my method. I won't have anyone coming to monitor my experiments".

Louis Pasteur

However the powers that be had decided, the theories of Pasteur were to be extolled and promoted, germs were the new public enemies and governments were to invest in techniques for their eradication.

CHAPTER 3 - SUMMARY

> ➤ Ideas of germ theory were developing in Europe during 19th century but had originated many years before

> ➤ The more accurate description of disease prevalent then, as judged by what we know today was developed by Antoine Béchamp

> ➤ Béchamp and others like him acknowledged that germs lived in the vast eco-system of the human body and diseases occurred due to toxic imbalances

> ➤ Pasteur however promoted the idea that germs alone were responsible for infectious disease, which allowed the public, commerce and government to avoid looking at the living conditions that promoted disease

> ➤ Germ theory satisfies a psychological, commercial and political agenda

CHAPTER FOUR

4 Pasteur's Germ Theory Revised - Based on What We Know Now

An up to date understanding about the role that germs (i.e. bacteria, fungi and viruses) play in health and disease

The ideas of Pasteur still dominant in the public perception of illness and equally pronounced in the orthodox treatment of disease do however need to be radically revised given the more up to date findings in microbiology. The Pasteur idea that microbes exist as externalised enemies requiring identification and eradication is of course a simple concept that does not account for the fact that human beings and in fact most multi-cellular beings live in partnership with large colonies of microbes in and around their bodies. Béchamp was in fact much closer to the truth than Pasteur.

Within the human body, there are trillions of microbes; they live in a 'symbiotic' relationship with each one of us. A symbiotic relationship is one where the microbe and the host live in <u>mutual benefit</u>; in fact they are often dependent on each other for survival, (as distinct from a parasitic relationship wherein a parasite lives at the expense of the host. Here of course the host does not benefit but often supports the parasite to the detriment of itself).

Microbes within the human body are necessary for your health, Dr Gibson, Food Microbial Sciences Unit, at The University of Reading, UK in 1996 states that …

> …" *There is much variability in bacterial numbers and populations between the stomach small intestine and colon. In comparison to other regions of the gastrointestinal tract, the human colon is an extremely densely populated microbial ecosystem - with the resident microbes representing around 95% of <u>all cells in the body</u>. The large gut flora is now accepted as playing a major role in both human pathogenesis and health - with the colon being the body's most metabolically active organ. Through diet, the composition of this microbial ecosystem can be influenced such that micro-organisms which are benign or health promoting can he stimulated.*"

These microbes carry out vital health functions in producing essential nutrients, aid in digestion and keep down levels of other potentially harmful microbes; however, these same microbes that are essential for health could equally become pathogenic (cause symptoms of disease) if conditions were to change; conditions that are influenced by, nutrition, toxins, enzyme levels, acidity, hormone levels, physical injury, emotional trauma, etc.

Therefore, many 'infections' can be more accurately described as 'imbalances' or even seen as positive symptoms of 'rebalancing' and are the <u>result</u> of the bodily conditions supporting these microbes. The microbes would have almost always been present prior to the onset of illness. Therefore it appears that microbes are the <u>result</u> of disease conditions and <u>not</u> the primary cause. REMEMBER here the context of this statement of microbes; the alternative to germ theory is that although microbes are involved in illness they did do not create the diseased condition of the patient in the first place, the diseased condition came first and produced the conditions for the microbes to multiply.

REMEMBER also that it appears as though microbes can pass from person to person but will only manifest disease in those that are susceptible and therefore produces a wide variety of symptoms from none, to more severe, to even death. Flu is a good example of an illness with a variety of symptoms that can occur at a certain time of year (e.g. in the winter when the temperature drops, sunlight reduces, and vitamin D levels diminish, to name a few issues) all of which may be associated with the same flu and therefore the same microbe, which are associated with no symptoms in most, some in others, severe in a few and even death in a tiny fraction, and yet in reality flu viruses are with us all the year round.

Finally REMEMBER that different microbes have their home in specific parts of the body and that true infection i.e. movement of microbes already within the body, to other parts of the body, can occur as a result of injury or disease. For example the movement of bacteria from colon to blood and then to the nervous system, as a result of the breakdown of the immune system and external membranes, could lead to septicaemia and meningitis. These microbes did not newly infect the patient but are, existing and necessary, microbes that are always present, but have been allowed to invade the interior of the patient as a 'result' of disease. We all have microbes on the membranes of our body capable of causing septicaemia and meningitis.

4.1 Bacteria - a necessary fact of life

Of the billions of microbes within the human body a large percentage of them occupy the spaces in contact with your mucous membranes and external skin, most appear to be external to your body fluids. Therefore although elements are in the digestive, urinary and respiratory tracts, they are essentially, as previously defined, outside of the body.

If you imagine the total number of cells in your entire body (estimated at around 50 to 100,000,000,000,000) then the number of **microbes** within the human body would be 10 times greater than the number of your own cells, of which **90% are in the digestive tract**. (The Lancet Vol. 361, Feb 08, 2003)

The microbes in the digestive tract are collectively known as the gut flora, and have many functions:

> Resist colonization of disease causing bacteria and fungus from our normal environment.
> Digestion of residues from the upper intestines that we are unable to digest with our own enzymes.
> Salvage of energy by producing short chain fatty acids for use by the body.
> Production of vitamins for the body
> Aid mineral absorption.
> Stimulate normal growth of intestinal cells (laboratory studies show they can also revert cancer growth)

The gut microbes represent the larger fraction of our microbial friends but there are of course more on the membranes of other tissues; the lungs, ears, nose, throat, genitourinary tracts and our skin. It is also known that these microbes can change their form, under toxic conditions and may produce additional bacterial toxic waste, in an already toxic environment. Bacteria are known to decompose dead tissue but do not 'attack' living tissue, as is often implied by our concept of disease-causing germs. We live in a symbiotic relationship with our microbes; part of a necessary ecosystem of the normal functioning healthy body.

4.2 Bacteria and the immune system in partnership

Recent research published in Public Library of Science (PLoS) Pathogens 22/07/2005, has also shown that bacteria not only regulate the numbers of other microbes by competing for space and resources but are able reduce opposing numbers by **working with the immune cells of the human body**. Literally calling in white blood cells (in this instance the white blood cells are neutrophils) to eradicate competing bacteria, researchers at the University Of Pennsylvania School Of Medicine studying two strains of bacteria normally present in the upper respiratory tract, found that one strain H. influenzae would attract white blood cells to kill off its rival S. pneumoniae.

> *"The results of this study show that recognition of microbial products from one species may activate inflammatory responses that promote the clearance of another competing species. This study also demonstrates how manipulations such as antibiotics or vaccines, which are meant to diminish the presence of a single pathogen, may inadvertently alter the competitive interactions of complex microbial communities."*

The results are being used to explain the side-effects of the pneumonia vaccine that is resulting in more middle ear infections.

4.3 Microbes changing form

There are many scientists since the 1900s; Dr Gunther Enderlein; Dr Rife, Dr Gaston Naessens, Dr Wilhelm Reich that have observed and demonstrated the ability of microbes to change form dramatically; changing into various types of bacteria and to fungal colonies and even creating viral particles.

Scientists working with live blood samples, using what is called 'dark field' or 'dark phase' microscopy, are able to observe microbes changing into these different forms according to the nature of their environment; the more acidic, the less oxygenated and the more polluted the bodily fluid, the more we find associated microbes. As acidity and toxicity levels increase and oxygen concentrations decrease these microbes grow larger and accumulate protein reserves as an adaptation to their environment and practitioners are able to remedy diseases and reduce these microbial populations by addressing the conditions that created the internal toxicity.

This ability of microbes to exhibit such extreme morphological change is called 'pleomorphism' and has historically been rejected by the orthodox medical establishment, although conventional scientists have more recently recognised many instances of pleomorphism. In addition, as published in the Journal of Clinical Microbiology, August 16 2002, conventional microbiological methods, have demonstrated the existence of populations of pleomorphic bacteria in healthy human blood, the internal fluid of the body that was always thought to be sterile in healthy individuals.

4.3.1 Dr Ryke Geerd Hamer

Additionally in the resolution of cancer tumours, many researchers have found that they often contain bacteria, and different tumours are consistently associated with different types of bacteria. Dr Ryke Geerd Hamer has an exceptionally high success rate with his cancer therapy; the public prosecutor's office of Wiener Neustadt examined 6500 patient cases from Burgau, who were considered incurable by traditional medical standards. Surprisingly, over 90% of these patients had survived, i.e. over 6000 using the methods of Dr Hamer. He has noted the presence of bacteria in tumour cells that have the function of destroying and digesting the tumour as an integral part of the healing response to cancer.

Dr Hamer's observations are being used by large numbers of practitioners; he has also demonstrated that significant emotional traumas will be interpreted by the patient in a way that reflects their own specific sensitivities and fears. He has distinguished four main types of emotional susceptibilities; separation, fear of survival, fear of attack and self-devaluation, each will impact on a specific part of the body and will have a corresponding impact in the brain as seen with an MRI scan.

The brain part affected will be reflective of the developmental tissue layer in embryology and will therefore correspond exactly to the appropriate part of the body. Thereby body-part, brain and emotion are exactly correlated and the role of the microbe is not seen as an indiscriminate agent, attacking the body, but an integral part of its healing mechanism in the breakdown of specific diseased tissue.

These facts are however still largely ignored by the present orthodoxy in terms of their practical approach to treating disease, mainly because they appear to undermine their own perspective and approach to treating illness. Orthodox interpretations tend to think of microbes as static elements unable to change form, known as monomorphism, and that pathogenic microbes are either present or not and that healthy human blood is sterile and therefore free of microbes. Consequently the way to deal with illness and the associated microbes, is simply to kill them.

There are of course major consequences to accepting the existence of microbes in healthy human blood and the phenomena of pleomorphism:

> Firstly the nature of the 'terrain' i.e. the body fluids, influences the nature and amount of microbe present, therefore it is much more imperative to address the nature of the terrain, determined by, diet, toxins and lifestyle, etc. as opposed to merely killing microbes.

> Secondly, according to the research of dark field microscopists, many of these microbes already exist within the blood, therefore not only do we have a widely accepted source of good bacteria and others associated with disease on our skin and mucous membranes (i.e. on the outside spaces of the body), the implication is that they can potentially exist on the inside, in places of the body that we previously thought were

'sterile', (i.e. containing no microbes at all – in particular bacteria).

➢ These bacteria exist in symbiotic balance with each other and in close relationship to the immune system; killing off some microbes will have wider implications, unintentionally compromising others and the functioning of the immune system.

➢ Thirdly, these microbes, like those that have been found in cancer tumours, are thought to have the ability to digest surrounding toxins, and dead tissue and thereby can be **an aid to immune function** rather than the primary cause of disease.

4.4 Antibiotics in principle – what happens when you kill off bacteria with antibiotics, i.e. without addressing the terrain?

With the proliferation of bacteria in diseased patients, antimicrobials may help to destroy microbes and thus slow down the cleanup process, creating some time for the human body to address toxic and microbial imbalances, they could certainly create some respite from microbial toxins. They may also be useful, especially as a last resort, when innate healing systems appear to be overloaded and in cases where microbes have infected the internal systems from the skin and mucous membranes from injuries and immune damage. But there are some potential problems with the use of antimicrobials that need to be factored in when designing protocols for managing disease.

Firstly, it is recognised within orthodox medicine that the elimination of bacteria by the use of antibiotics as a first resort does not allow the immune system to develop its own natural ability to deal with such imbalances.

Secondly, antibiotics will destroy many of the bacteria that are important for health and this upsets the balance of healthy bacteria within the body and can predispose the patient to other opportunistic bacteria or fungus, exacerbating the situation. Fungal symptoms of thrush are a common consequence of antibiotic treatment.

This effect can have even more severe consequences in new born children. In the first days of life babies develop a tolerance to appropriate populations of beneficial bacteria, however, the use of antibiotics at this stage can increase the likelihood of microbes associated with illness colonising their digestive tracts on a more permanent basis, not just for the period whilst taking antibiotics. It has been demonstrated that such children can find it very difficult to maintain healthy populations of beneficial bacteria right into adulthood and are predisposed to digestive disturbances, inflammatory conditions, systemic fungal conditions, blood toxicity, neurological problems, allergies, colon cancer and whole host of related illnesses.

Thirdly, the microbial response to 'disease' rather than being the cause may in fact be part of the curative response and therefore the body's method of utilising microbes to digest dead tissue and toxins, killing these microbes will therefore have a detrimental effect on the patient, slowing down the clean-up process and prolonging the disease.

Fourthly, the antibiotic itself is a poisonous chemical that has to be detoxified by the liver etc and then eliminated from the body, this would then actually add to the problem if in fact we are already struggling with an overburdened immune system and increased toxic load.

In addition, if the predisposing factors of diet or toxic build-up from other sources are not addressed, then killing the pathogenic bacteria would only make way for the production of more pathogenic bacteria, produced from the vast pool of existing bacteria within the system.

If antibiotics have been used, then the least resistant strains are killed first, leaving a certain number of the most resistant strains surviving. This is why we are asked to finish a course of antibiotics; to kill off all the last remaining, and most resistant strains. However, this is an empty rhetoric; there will <u>always</u> be some survivors and so long as the predisposing factors are not dealt with, then these microbes along with any predecessors to pathogenic bacteria will then create the new dominant forms of bacteria.

These forms will be resistant to the initial antibiotic and so a new antibiotic will be needed. This cycle of administering antibiotics, leaving the most resistant strains left, can continue until the predominant surviving bacteria are resistant to all the known forms of antibiotic and we would have created the 'superbug'.

This so-called super-bug is no more capable of creating symptoms of illness than any other bug, it just happens to be resistant to our antibiotics. If the predisposing factors are not addressed then these bacteria will dominate and proliferate contributing to the consequences of disease. Because many holistic practitioners do not give antibiotics and prefer instead to address the conditions that cause and maintain these microbes, then illnesses associated with so-called super-bugs can be treated just as easily as any other condition involving other microbes.

The superbug is <u>not</u> a consequence of unclean hospitals and treatment centres, they may be spread because of poor cleanliness but they are formed by the overuse of antibiotics and in fact they tend to be most common in the cleanest parts of hospitals; intensive care units, surgical wards and operating theatres. They are a direct consequence of antibiotic treatment with the concomitant disregard of the causative factors of the illness.

It is possible that after the use of antibiotics, the human body can redress the toxic imbalance; eliminating toxins through vomiting, diarrhoea, mucus discharge, fasting through natural loss of appetite, bed rest, inflammatory responses etc. Antibiotics can slow this down and so appear to give you time, and may be useful as a last resort, however, unless the underlying toxicity issues have been addressed then the antibiotic is ultimately useless, microbes will continue to grow and prolonged use of antibiotics may eventually create more problems than they solve.

4.5 The role of viruses in disease.

Having made the assumption that inflammatory reactions, the formation of rashes and the production of mucus and other discharges were the definitive signs of 'infection', scientists then discovered that exactly those symptoms could be produced without bacteria.

Before modern scientific techniques were able to isolate, characterise and photograph minute particles, it was initially inferred that these illnesses were caused by microscopic elements called viruses, which eventually lead to the search and characterisation for these new pathogens. These viruses quickly became the new physiological enemy, the definitive bio-terrorist, and many so-called infectious illnesses were defined by the specific virus that were thought to be the cause of the illness; measles, rubella, chickenpox, AIDS, polio, etc.

However the issue of viral causation in disease is far from clear; remember that Koch defined the basic criteria by which scientists could determine whether an illness could be defined as being caused by a microbe (mainly for bacteria and protozoa single-cell organisms).

> The bacteria must be present in every case of the disease.

> ➢ The bacteria must be isolated from the host with the disease and grown in pure culture.
> ➢ The specific disease must be reproduced when a pure culture of the bacteria is inoculated into a healthy susceptible host.

These Koch's Postulates were however redefined in 1937 and 1982 in an attempt to accommodate the new diseases that were thought to be caused by viruses.

Redefined because, many viruses could easily exist in humans that do not cause disease; many could not be isolated and identified in cases of disease; many isolated viruses could not reproduce the illness through skin contact, breathed in or ingested through the digestive tract but only if injected in large quantities directly into the body, which of course is not the method by which most of these illnesses are contracted. The viral theory of disease has many exceptions and anomalies.

4.6 What are viruses?

Does your doctor know what a virus is and what it does?

Viruses are effectively small packets of genes, chemically composed of DNA or RNA. Genes are the information that the cell uses to reproduce exact copies of itself and they also provide a blue-print for the production of proteins that determine the structure and function of each cell. A virus is a very small amount of this genetic material covered in a protective coat, viruses are much smaller than bacteria and although we talk of 'live vaccines' implying the virus is still alive, viruses themselves are not living things. 'Live' from the point of view of vaccine manufacturers really means 'not destroyed' or 'not chemically annihilated' or not a genetically engineered chemical copy.

A virus contains **only** genetic information and has no other elements capable of digesting, eliminating, reproducing, moving, etc. It can carry out **none** of the functions requisite for life; a virus is basically a sophisticated chemical. However, the genetic information from the virus can be taken in by a host cell and in some instances they can be reproduced by that host cell producing more viral copies. There are in fact many kinds of viruses in almost all forms of life; plants, animals and bacteria.

The controversy lies in the significance of viruses in disease and therefore the **viral disease theory**. As with other microbes, we have been told that:

> The virus is the cause of many viral illnesses and can only infect from outside of the host or cell. Once within the host cell, the host reproduces the virus in great number, very rapidly, (the virus is not capable of doing this on its own), and consequently the host cell dies, bursts open and releases many more viruses into the tissue of the body, whereupon they are able to infect more cells. These infected cells are then hijacked to reproduce more viruses in the same manner as before, thereby causing symptoms of disease and in severe cases the eventual death of the host.

However, there are considerable problems with this theory, problems that in many ways mirror the situation with bacteria.

> ➢ Most viruses that infect bacteria, plants, and animals (including humans) do not cause disease. In fact, scientists have studied viruses at length and have found those that infect bacteria may be helpful, in that they rapidly transfer genetic information from

one bacterium to another. Viruses of plants and animals may convey genetic information among similar species, aiding the survival of their hosts in hostile environments.

Encyclopaedia Britannica, Macropaedia (1990) p507:
Recited in "Images of Polio" – by Jim West

➤ This method of acquiring genes is not in doubt. Bacteria as well as higher animal cells including humans are known to acquire viral genes, and the phenomenon is not rare. Endogenous viruses and viral elements have been found in all vertebrates investigated. As a general rule, the number of groups of viral sequences found within a given vertebrate species is proportional to the effort spent searching that species, i.e. whenever we look we find them and the more we look the more we find.

➤ The supposed AIDS virus (HIV) is said to be responsible for the immune breakdown of a patient with symptoms of AIDS, by the insertion of viral genetic information into the T-cells of the patient's DNA (genes). It is very difficult to conceive how such a small amount of nucleic acid that is supposed to be found in only 1% of T-cells can account for the range of pathology seen in AIDS. Recently it has become known that approximately 3,000 times that amount of viral DNA already exists in normal cells. (Eleni Papadopulos-Eleopulos, in Continuum, Autumn 1997). The connection between AIDS and HIV is extremely controversial many of the original researchers <u>do not</u> even accept that the virus HIV is responsible for AIDS.

➤ Scientists have also demonstrated the ability of **cells** to **produce viruses** when under threat from external poisons and radiation, it is known as the SOS response in bacteria. This is in fact part of the reaction to poisons that is a standard chemical test used in the pharmaceutical industry and agrochemical industry to assess the toxicity of additives, drugs and insecticides called the 'Ames' test. Such a phenomenon is almost completely unknown within the consciousness of the general public, the fact that under chemical stress cells will actually produce viruses.

> Cells producing viruses under such circumstances could be:

  o A method of informing or warning other cells of the danger

  o Instructing other cells how to affect the required response to the trauma, just as genetic resistance to antibiotics can be transferred to other bacteria in this manner.

  o The packaging of the DNA codes as with other cell components to be recycled and used by other cells as the cell faces destruction.

> Therefore, rather than the cause of cell breakdown, we know that viruses are caused by the poisoning of cells, the cell effectively breaks up and packages tiny amounts of its genetic material in protective membranes; these are in fact viruses. A poisoned cell effectively produces viruses and therefore it is very likely that the reason why so much viral DNA/RNA is found in normal cellular DNA is because that is where the viral DNA actually came from, viruses are in fact broken up pieces of our own cellular DNA.

> We also know that viruses transfer useful genetic information from cell to cell and to other individuals in <u>healthy</u> cells, yet surprisingly we have **never** been able to show a virus infecting a host cell from the outside to the inside creating a diseased cell. In the decades of viral research using electron microscopes able to detect small particles such as viruses, we have never been able to show what is known as 'infectosomes' in diseased cells, i.e. viruses being incorporated in the membrane of a host cell transferring genetic information into the cell causing its disease and destruction.

➢ All examples of supposed viral elements in disease seem to corroborate the fact that these elements are caused by poisoning cells first and that viruses are in fact the breakdown products of the cell. Dying cells will often breakdown internally, packaging up its molecular components in membrane bound portions. In programmed cell death this process is called apoptosis. The transfer of these supposed viruses to other cells although they can be incorporated in healthy cells does <u>not</u> subsequently create disease in those cells.

➢ Additionally, because the normal products of cells follow a line of activity from genes in the nucleus to outside of the nucleus, scientists naturally assumed that any 'back-flow' was pathological. There was an assumption that activity should not flow back into the nucleus affecting the genes. This 'Reverse Transcription' as it is called, was deemed pathology, a mal-function, a cause of disease, and was assumed to be caused by a virus that was changing the patients DNA or inserting its own viral DNA in the patient. However we have since learnt that this activity often occurs when the cell is carrying out normal DNA repair, it is more likely to be occurring as a result of disease rather than causing a disease.

In fact the many illnesses that are diagnosed as viral have never had a positive identification of such; it is usually a diagnosis by default, if nothing else can be found then it's probably viral.

Expensive lab tests involve characterising the DNA of assumed viruses; this is rarely performed on patients that are ill. Very occasionally a clinical test for the antibodies to a virus is used which infers the presence of a virus but again this is subject to interpretation. There isn't a reliable clinical test for the viruses themselves, so the actual virus is not tested for, just the presence of antibodies to the virus. It is therefore highly probable that viruses may be present but with undetectable levels of antibody to them. As such, not only are there inherent problems in ascertaining whether a virus is the cause of an illness, but additional problems in ascertaining whether a virus is actually there or not and if it is present, whether it has 'infected' the host or always been there.

The HIV test is in fact a test for an antibody to a protein that has been assumed to be from the virus, but the virus has <u>never been isolated</u>. In addition most people will in fact test positive for the presence of this antibody, but there has been an agreed concentration of antibody that suddenly defines whether you are HIV positive or not. Below that concentration you are considered negative; above that you are considered positive, therefore this does <u>not</u> state that someone who is HIV positive has the antibody and someone who is HIV negative does not. Those testing negative could and often do have lower levels of these antibodies.

Dr Stefan Lanka a German research scientist having studied molecular biology and ecology started viral research in 1986. Then as the public became aware of AIDS and its connection with a virus (HIV), he was automatically considered an expert on AIDS. However when checking the literature of previous research on AIDS he found that scientists were not providing proof of a virus. Dr Lanka was deeply shocked but wanted to be sure…

"Well, I'm not experienced enough. I have overlooked something. On the other side, those people are absolutely sure. Then I was afraid that speaking about this with my friends, or even my family, they would think is absolutely mad and crazy. So for a long time I studied virology, from the end to the beginning, from the beginning to the end, to be absolutely sure that there was no such thing as HIV. And it was easy for me to be sure about this because I realized that the whole group of viruses to which HIV is said to belong, the retroviruses -- as well as other viruses which are claimed to be very dangerous -- in fact do not exist at all."…

"For almost one year we have been asking authorities, politicians and medical institutes after the scientific evidence for the existence of such viruses that are said to cause disease and therefore require "immunization". After almost one year we have not received even one concrete answer which provides evidence for the existence of those "vaccination viruses". The conclusion is inevitable that our children are still vaccinated on the basis of scientific standards of the 18th and 19th century. In the 19th century Robert Koch demanded in his generally accepted postulates evidence of the virus in order to prove infection; at Koch's time this evidence couldn't be achieved directly by visualization and characterization of the viruses, because adequate technology wasn't available at that time. Methods of modern medicine have profoundly changed over the past 60 years, in particular by the invention of the electron microscope. And still all these viruses we get immunized against have never been re-examined using this technology?"…

Regarding the available photographic proof of viruses studied by Dr Lanka:

"All these photos have in common that they, (the authors), can't claim that they present a virus, as long as they do not also provide the original publications which describe how and what from the virus has been isolated. Such original publications are cited **nowhere**. Indeed, in the entire scientific literature there's not even one publication, where "viruses in the disease" the fulfilment of Koch's first postulate is even claimed. That means that there is no proof that from humans with certain diseases the viruses - which are held responsible for these diseases - have been isolated. Nevertheless, this is precisely what they publicly claim."

www.klein-klein-aktion.de

The role of microbes as causative agents of disease is indeed sketchy; in fact techniques in most of the alternative therapies have focussed on detoxification, immune building, adding friendly bacteria and working with the elimination procedures of the body, etc. None of which have ever required a positive identification of a microbe that has needed to be killed.

Summary

Let us now be clear about these issues, bacteria and fungus are living micro-organisms (unlike viruses), what is in question is their role in the 'causation' of disease, and more particularly infectious disease. Bacteria and fungus can be utilised by the body to digest toxins even though this process of digestion can produce other toxic by-products some of which ca also cause symptoms, the disease causation would have been the initial toxicity and cellular breakdown. As such you cannot catch these diseases from someone else unless your cellular environment is the same as the next person, in which case you are reacting to your circumstances eliminating toxins, and thereby cultivating microbes, not catching microbes that have caused your disease.

Bacteria and fungus can also contaminate the body from an external source if for example you were to ingest decayed and contaminated food which would add to your toxicity; as such we have an issue of food/water poisoning, not an infectious disease, even if you could irradiate and kill microbes from such contaminated food the food quality itself would still cause illness because it is no longer nutritious but poisonous.

Additionally, an injury to one part of our body can allow microbes to enter and therefore contaminate other parts of our body that are ordinarily relatively microbe free, thus causing symptoms of disease, again this is a special case caused by injury and not an infectious disease.

Viruses on the other hand are not living microbes, they have not been demonstrated as the cause of disease, they are mostly present in stable relationships with certain host cells and have only been isolated, characterised and electron-micrographed (i.e. photographed) in primitive cells.

Rather than a demonstrable cause of disease, viruses have been verified as being caused by the poisoning of cells and have never been found to infect cells in disease tissue, furthermore none have ever been characterised by the techniques currently available in modern virology. Their presence is by inference by indirect supposition but what is particularly damning is that the technology to isolate, characterise and electron micrograph viruses is in fact now readily available but has so far not been able to demonstrate the presence or causation of viruses in disease tissue.

The viral story is quite an incredible tale going back to the days of Edward Jenner and the imagined smallpox virus to the present day, with virus classifications apparently based on membrane proteins, enzymes and genetic material. But here the perspective of virologist Stefan Lanka is quite instructive, he shows how in fact the viral disease theories are based on belief systems creating hypothesis, leading to assumption and more supposition, inferred from very limited biological experiments, none of which has been verified using the techniques we now have available in modern science.

> *If ever a virus coming from a specific body or a body fluid, for instance from birds, has been proven, then any average scientist can verify, in any average laboratory, within a day, whether this virus is present in for instance a dead animal. This has however never occurred, and on the contrary, indirect test methods which tell absolutely nothing are being used.*
>
> **Stefan Lanka**

How do they know that viruses are present in disease?

4.6.1 Viral anti-bodies

In trying to assess if a given virus is present scientists test the body for antibodies produced in response to the virus. However, these antibody tests are not specific, antibodies can be produced by the body in response to a range of particles not just one virus, finding antibodies in an individual is supposed to demonstrate that the virus was present but these antibodies may have been produced in response to other things. Therefore the presence of, for example, measles antibody does NOT tell you that measles virus is necessarily present, which is how these tests can produce false positives. In addition even if these tests were accurate, antibodies to viruses do not inform whether the virus is the cause of the disease, just that the viral particle was present.

4.6.2 Viral DNA/RNA testing

Testing for viral DNA has not been carried out by isolating the virus first, (which remember we do have techniques for doing) instead pieces of DNA found in the diseased cells or fluids are multiplied up, using biochemical techniques called polymerase chain reactions. This DNA could in fact be from anywhere in the body and is never verified by comparing to real viral DNA because the real viruses in diseases have never been isolated. With no standard viral isolation we have no way of verifying whether theses multiplied pieces of DNA are from virus or not.

4.6.3 Viral properties

Other biochemical properties of the virus are again assumed by taking the disease fluid and adding that to cells, which may cause, for example, cells to stick to each other (e.g. haemagglutinin). This is assumed to be the way the virus sticks to a cell and enters cells causing the illness. But again even though we have all kinds of elaborate hypotheses as to how this viral sticking occurs, we have never isolated these cells undergoing attachment and infection, and never photographed them using modern electron microscopy techniques.

Other reactions caused by enzymes in these disease fluids are again inferred as viral, for example neuraminidase reactions are said to be from the virus, but again these enzymes are common products of immune cells, for example in the lysosomal parts of the body's own white blood cells that are used to break down unwanted cell debris, poisons, and microbes.

4.6.4 What about Antiviral medication – How can the help if many viruses don't cause diseases?

Some drugs that are used to counteract the action of viruses (anti-virals) are in fact just neuraminidase inhibitors, which supposedly; reduce cell breakdown, viral entry and therefore viral replication. However recent research shows how neuraminidase activity actually enhances our own cellular immune activity, therefore anti-retrovirals thought to be inhibiting the virus may just be simple immune suppressors inhibiting our own immune cells. Suppressing our immune reactions with drugs will usually give initial relief but in the long-term reduces the body's ability to deal with the problem.

> "...the results of the current study clearly indicate a slowdown influence of neuraminidase on apoptosis in peripheral blood lymphocytes. The study shows that neuraminidase decreased the level of apoptosis in blood lymphocytes and **increased their vitality**."

Journal of Physiology & Pharmacology, 2007 (58) Suppl 5, 253-262

That is to say if neuraminidase increases our immune cell activity then anti-neuraminidase drugs (so-called anti-virals) will slow down our immune cell activity.

A web site publicising these issues www.klein-klein-aktion.de has been set up by an organisation in Germany, pushing health authorities to acknowledge the lack of scientific confirmation of these viral disease theories, their experience has been quite illuminating:

> "We have sent our questions to the Health Officials, Social Ministers of the German states, University clinics, local Doctors groups, Federal Doctor groups, the Robert-Koch-Institute, the Paul-Ehrlich-Institute, Research establishments and the Health Ministry in Bonn. In our desperation we have also turned to many Public Health politicians, to the State parliaments of Baden Wurttemberg and Bavaria, to the Federal parliament and to the Chancellor's office. We have requested the Press for help. We have requested Doctors for help. We still haven't received a single clear answer to our specific questions.

> ...The authorities refer to the evidence of a time in which the virus couldn't be isolated, presented, characterised and photographed because the necessary technology wasn't developed. Viruses were diagnosed on the basis of symptoms. One can reasonably guess from this that the concept Contagion = poison = virus from the 18th & 19th centuries was transferred onto the components of cells which in the 20th century are referred to as a virus. The astonishing thing is that these descriptions apparently emerge in the secondary literature and are drawn upon as an explanation for poisoning and vaccine damage.

> ...Although Professor Forschepiepe and Dr Buchwald first made this proposal to the Ministry for Health and Hygiene in Bonn in 1961. Since then the authorities have provided us with hundreds of so-called "Virus pictures". The Biologists and micro-biologists to whom we have presented these pictures, have adjudicated that in every case these viruses are not characterised and isolated. Certainly these pictures concern cellular tissue-thin-sections and cellular tissue-cross-sections."

In summary, many kinds of laboratory tests can infer the presence of disease, for example, there are tests that will show the presence of 'prostate specific antigen' (PSA) which can be indicative of prostate cancer, but other proteins could give a false positive and there may be other reasons for the presence of PSA, therefore once we have that test result it is then imperative that we go back to the patient and look at his prostate to confirm whether or not there is a tumour. This is of course exactly what happens in cancer diagnosis, however the problem with viral research is that we have the 'inference' i.e. lots of tests to show what viruses could do, but the verification has been omitted; nobody is going back to isolate and electron micrograph the virus. Initially this was because we simply didn't have the technology but now we do, is it avoided because we could be opening up a veritable can of worms …or a can of nothing?

The implication of the microbe from the point of view of Body Intelligence

The concept of body intelligence in disease recognises that symptoms of disease are intelligent reactions of the body when stressed beyond its normal limits. For example ingested poisons in food could cause nausea and vomiting, therefore in creating health and avoiding disease it is important to understand and distinguish the problem (ingested poisons) from the reaction to the problem (nausea and vomiting).

In addition because the human body is approximately 90% microbial cells in number it is significant also to understand that these microbes help in the normal functioning of the body and may also help to clean the body of poisons and dead cells when in disease.

The microbial population of the body responds to the environment, just as our own cells do, microbes are not opponents, intent on killing its host body i.e. us, but live harmoniously among our own cells, striving for the optimum health of its host. Even the newer bio-terrorists, viruses, are not the adversaries we once thought, most viruses studied are found to be useful, live in harmony with host cells and are not associated with diseases. They can be produced in great numbers as a result of poisoning cells and so reflect the toxicity of our environment and are therefore not causative of these conditions. Understanding the relationship of microbial populations to each other and to our own cells enables us to see the true nature of disease; the environmental conditions in which we place ourselves.

Current concepts of so-called infectious disease from an orthodox perspective view symptoms as malfunctions caused by the microbial enemy, they focus on the inability of the body to combat these attacking microbes which therefore require the ingestion of drugs to kill them. This concept of disease once again completely disregards the susceptibility of the host, the person in which the microbe lives, most individuals with these bacteria, fungus or virus do not succumb to symptoms of disease, by trying to kill microbes the real reasons as to what makes someone susceptible to illness are not addressed.

The patient is encouraged to fear microbes and ignore environmental causes of disease, creating a subtle power shift from patient to doctor, to drug, to Pharmaceutical Corporation, removing the significance of the impact of a deteriorating environment on our health.

As such we lose the ability to understand the true intelligence of the healing body, as well as the beneficent nature of our microbial partners.

CHAPTER 4 - SUMMARY

> Current research in microbiology demonstrates that the human being is a vast eco-system of its own human cells and microbes, (bacteria, fungus and viruses). Approximately ten times the number of cells in the body are microbes; there are more cells in your body that are not you, than are you.

> The internal environments of the body, including the microbes living within you, are affected by ingested toxins, nutrition, drugs, stress and hormones.

> Diseases associated with microbes are dependent on the susceptibility (the internal environment) of the person, because invading microbes are associated with illness in only a small percentage of people.

> Microbes are more often than not beneficial even during symptoms of disease.

> Disease symptoms are intelligent reactions to a stressed body reflected in environmental conditions and/or certain lifestyle choices.

CHAPTER FIVE

5 Treating Symptoms of 'Dis-ease'

The consequences of suppressing symptoms with medication, the immediate impact on the body and the resulting susceptibility to illnesses in the future

We have so far established that our toxins are eliminated by the normal everyday functions of the body; defecation, urination, perspiration and respiration. If toxins build at a greater rate than we are capable of eliminating them, then we experience symptoms of illness whereby the body increases the physical elimination of toxins and associated microbes including bacteria, fungus and viruses by:

- Vomiting and diarrhoea.
- Respiratory mucus with coughing, sneezing and nasal discharge.
- Increased sweating and urination, with increased concentration and odour.

We are aware that this situation has not been directly 'caused' by the microbe and that therefore illnesses being described as infectious illnesses are misleading as to the real causes of disease. The response to increased toxins, with an increase in physical elimination, may also involve white blood cells in the mucus; these specialised immune cells are able to break down toxins and associated microbes that have accumulated as a result of the increased toxicity.

It is important to realise that these symptoms are <u>not</u> physiological malfunctions but they are precise coordinated responses to a build-up of toxicity and a subsequent imbalance of microbes. Most of the holistic therapies are able to perceive the bigger picture. By taking a step back and including all the functions and symptoms of the individual, they are able to understand the purpose of symptoms. Therefore we shall revisit the question...

> *"Should we treat the symptoms of disease, or are they an aid to recovery?"*
>
> **The New Scientist, Oct 23, 1993**

5.1 Cured or suppressed

Realising that the symptoms of illness perform a necessary function for our survival, we arrive at one of the most significant elements in our understanding of health, illness and the treatment of disease. Using this example of toxicity; now that we appreciate how increased levels of toxicity within the digestive system would lead to an elimination response e.g. vomiting and/or diarrhoea, we are able to distinguish 'the response', (the vomiting and diarrhoea), from 'the problem', (the toxins).

In orthodox medicine often the response itself is seen as the problem and the real causes are frequently ignored; we visit our doctor with the problem of vomiting and diarrhoea. From this perspective we would be tempted to try and stop the reaction, believing that the vomiting and diarrhoea are themselves the problems to be stopped. Many pharmaceutical drugs are designed to do just that and the sales of such drugs to the public and to health authorities, hinge on that basic premise. Selling more drugs relies on the ability to maintain the perspective that the symptom is a mal-function. Whilst we are convinced the symptom is the problem (rather than indicative of a problem) then the solution lies in drug intervention capable of stopping the perceived problem.

As obvious as it may seem, this New Scientist commentary helps us to acknowledge this current medical omission.

> *"The underlying message is uncontroversial enough: human beings and their illnesses are the products of a long evolutionary history. Yet <u>modern medicine</u>, for all its high-technology treatments and preventive strategies, <u>has so far largely ignored this fact</u>."*
>
> **The New Scientist, Oct 23, 1993**

So with the build-up of toxins in the digestive tract leading to vomiting and diarrhoea we may be given an anti-emetic to stop the vomiting and Imodium to stop the diarrhoea. However, from our wider perspective, knowing that the 'symptom' is a 'response' to the problem of intestinal toxicity, taking something to stop the reaction is **'suppressive'**. The symptoms may have been stopped but the problem is not resolved and one of the central themes of a holistic approach to health care is the understanding of this concept of **suppression**.

We could, however, justify the uses of suppressive medication if we were concerned about the effects of our responses; the response itself could be extremely uncomfortable, the response could persist for too long and it may also lead to secondary complications. For example excessive vomiting and diarrhoea could lead to dehydration with subsequent loss of other functions, in addition to headaches, low blood pressure, electrolyte imbalance etc.

All of which are valid concerns, which would therefore lead us to addressing these issues, treatment from your health practitioner would be successful according to their understanding of the illness. We would have to address the problem of the build-up of toxicity, perhaps stimulate the elimination response and at the same time support the general function by re-hydrating, replacing minerals etc.

However, without a perspective of the purpose of the response and knowledge of the possibility of suppression, doctors are likely to suppress all responses without distinguishing which of them is a necessary part of the curative response. Suppressing vitally important reactions could of course lead to more severe consequences.

> *"Most diseases are the result of medication which has been prescribed to relieve and take away a beneficent and warning symptom on the part of Nature."*
>
> **Elbert Hubbard (19/06/1856 – 7/05/ 1915)**
> **American writer, publisher, artist, and philosopher**

In fact the pharmaceutical intervention of physiological responses in that manner is really only justified in 'end-state' pathology, when in fact the patient is unable to react, or when the reactions have become detrimental to the patient, the medical profession does in fact excel in accident and emergency situations. However it is an unfortunate fact of orthodox medical intervention that they have taken the rationale for treating emergency situations, to treat virtually all other conditions.

With our example of toxicity within the digestive tract leading to vomiting and diarrhoea, suppression of the actual response would in fact increase the chances of an '**unsuccessful**' elimination reaction and could therefore result in the very situation we are trying to avoid, recurrent symptoms and/or prolonged symptoms.

> **Pharmaceutical suppression increases the chances of the ultimate symptom scenario many doctors say they are trying to avoid.**

5.2 Consequences of Suppression

From our example of toxic build-up within the digestive tract and subsequent response of vomiting and diarrhoea, we may ask, what happens to our problem after effective suppression of our response?

What happens to those toxins that we have been trying to eliminate with the vomiting and diarrhoea if we suppress the vomiting and diarrhoea? Quite clearly, these toxins can remain; attracting germs (microbes) and changing the nature of the germs that are normally present. With these microbes and toxins remaining within the digestive tract, they could poison the tissues and cells in that region of the body. Toxins may even build up and pass across the membrane of the digestive tract into the blood system where they would then have access to other internal organs.

The suppression of the body's attempt to 'eliminate', could therefore lead to more serious and/or more internal problems. To avoid this, the body's immune system will once again react, leading to either a recurrence of the vomiting and diarrhoea or will engage other systems in an attempt to detoxify, eliminate or limit the damage caused by these potential poisons.

5.2.1 Asthma and suppressive medication

The relevance of suppression in the deterioration of health is particularly striking when considering the incidence and deaths due to asthma. Until the 1950's asthma was not considered to be life threatening, however, more recently according to the CDC in the United States, rates of death due to asthma have risen 42% in the period between 1982 and 1992, and asthma has increased by 52% in persons between the ages of 5 and 34. A more recent study by the CDC indicates that asthma has doubled during the last 20 years and is now the most common disorder in children and adolescents.

Research by Michel Odent reported in the Journal of the American Medical Association (1994; 272:592-3) showed that the use of whooping cough vaccine increased the incidence of asthma by 5-6 times as compared to non-vaccinated children. This was later confirmed by research at Churchill Hospital in Oxford UK and presented to the British Thoracic Society by Chest Consultant, Dr Julian Hopkin.

People with asthma experience a tightening of the chest and constriction of the bronchioles (the lung tubes), the sensation can be distressing and these uncomfortable symptoms of asthma were seen as the primary problems to be solved.

An article in 'What Doctors Don't Tell You' (Vol. 4 No. 6 1993) gave an account of Dr John Mansfield (President of the British Society of Allergy and Environmental Medicine) and Dr David Freed (Formerly lecturer in immunology, Manchester University) regarding the treatment of asthma:

Beta agonists were a class of drugs given to help widen the tubes of the lungs during an asthma attack. The use of these drugs was thought to be dangerous and therefore in the mid-1960's drug consumption fell along with death rate. However, as reported in Recent advances in Respiratory Medicine (4: 1986; 1-11), by the mid 1970's as confidence again grew in what were thought to be safer bronchodilators, prescription rates increased along with death rates.

It appears that when the lungs are in crisis and need to eliminate toxins, the tubes of the lungs naturally narrow thus increasing the pressure of air through them, together with the coughing reflex this enables the mucus and other debris to be pushed and scoured out through the lung tubes. This toxin and debris elimination by the process of coughing is much more difficult, if not impossible, if the lung tubes remain open or are forced open by the use of drugs.

Asthma deaths were often thought to be due to under diagnosis, asthma we are told is a more dangerous condition than the public are aware of and deaths were due to insufficient medical treatment. However post mortem investigations revealed otherwise, two types of asthmatic conditions were discovered and in fact the most common being in individuals with a history of increasingly aggressive medical treatment rather than insufficient treatment. Examination of their lungs after death revealed that their airways were plugged with mucus so thick and hard that it could not be sucked up with the normal pipettes but had to be scraped out with a knife. This is in fact a direct consequence of drugs that are used to force open the lung tubes during asthma. It is therefore not the side-effects of the drugs that are dangerous but the actual primary effect of the drug. The drug is working against the natural responses of the body, stopping the important tightening of the airways that enables the elimination of toxins and mucus.

This lead Mansfield and Freed to come to the conclusion that:

> *"It is the doctors who have turned asthma into a killer. Any drug, that effectively reverses constriction and inflammation of the airways, renders the patient more susceptible to the direct toxic effects of the particles and chemicals that the inflammation was trying to remove, and therefore is likely to increase mortality".*

CHAPTER 5 – SUMMARY

> ➤ There is a difference between the symptom reaction and the problem, stress or trauma
> ➤ Understanding the purpose of symptoms as attempts of the body to address the conditions of disease enables one to see the detrimental consequences of stopping those symptoms with medication
> ➤ Symptoms have a purpose and can therefore succeed or fail in that purpose
> ➤ Symptom suppression with medication increases the risk of a prolonged disease and increases the risk of more serious disease, affecting deeper and more important parts of the body
> ➤ Symptom suppression has a place in disease management where the patient is no longer able to respond to the problem and the symptoms themselves are creating additional problems
> ➤ The proportion of cases that really require suppression are a very small fraction of cases that currently undergo suppressive treatments

CHAPTER SIX

6 Your Illness – was it cured or does it remain unresolved?

Are some illnesses really an opportunity for the body to learn how to deal with stress beyond its current limits and therefore a path to improved health?

Once we have recognised that the response of the body to a problem is a necessary step to resolving the problem, we are able to understand the reactions of the human body in illness in a more holistic manner. Knowing the purpose of symptoms in disease, we can see beyond what appears to be an inconvenient and unnecessary discomfort.

It is immediately apparent that merely eliminating a symptom does not necessarily resolve our predicament; the end of an acute illness would therefore result in either a successful resolution of the problem or a failure to resolve the issue; failure would therefore leave us with an **unresolved** illness, here the nature of the symptoms may change or diminish, but they do not simply disappear, the patient is still unwell.

What factors determine whether acute illnesses resolve or not?

- A. The amount of trauma/stress that the patient is responding to.
- B. The reactive energy /vitality of the patient.
- C. The management of their symptoms; helping or suppressing.

A. The level of trauma imposed on the individual (the immediate reason for their symptoms)

The level of trauma: As regard to a physical injury, is fairly self-evident, the lower the level of trauma, the more likelihood of there being a successful response. With an acute infectious disease we are apt to believe that the level of trauma is determined by the virulence of the microbe or perhaps how many happen to be there. These, however, are not primarily relevant. For example the exact same microbe that could lead to the death of one individual is biologically identical to one that is tolerated and therefore produces no symptoms at all in another individual. With a so-called infectious illness the degree of trauma in this instance relates to the degree of toxicity of the patient, how toxic is the individual and therefore what and how many microbes are proliferating within their system. As we shall see later 'virulence' is actually a function of the patient, i.e. it is determined by the health of the patient, not the microbe.

B. The vitality of the individual: How much physical, mental and emotional energy does the individual have to react with.

The vitality, the reactive power of the individual is determined by the common primary health factors, nutritional status, oxygenation, rest, relaxation, sleep, physical energy, physical function, mental state, emotional feelings etc these are factors that determine the likelihood of a successful response to a trauma and therefore the reactive capacity of the individual.

C. How much of the reaction to the trauma is being suppressed.

Finally the management of the illness i.e. whether symptoms are helped or suppressed will critically determine the success or failure of the body in responding to trauma. From what we have so far discussed, it is apparent that if the body reacts to trauma, as you would experience in an acute disease, the suppression of that reaction would decrease the likelihood of a successful response, we can still sometimes succeed despite suppression but we are less likely to.

6.1 What are the possible outcomes of acute disease

As well as distinguishing the two most obvious results of disease; success and failure - we can further delineate another two. Thus we can envisage four approximate outcomes to an acute disease as follows:

1. The individual resolves the illness and as a result, the health is improved and they are stronger than they were before. They are then less susceptible to those problems after the illness and more able to deal with them.
2. The individual resolves the illness but there has been no learning as such, they are not stronger than they were before, they effectively carry on, as they were before the illness, just as susceptible to succumbing to the illness as they were before.
3. The illness is not resolved and as a result the health of the individual is worse than before and they descend into a lower level of chronic illness, more susceptible than before.
4. The illness is not resolved and the patient is unable to react sufficiently to overcome the problem and dies.

We can illustrate this diagrammatically as follows:

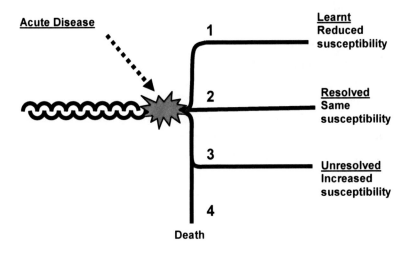

By returning to our example of toxicity in the digestive tract leading to the reaction of vomiting and diarrhoea, we can illustrate the above phenomena and see its significance in our daily life.

6.1.1 Resolution of illness leading to an increased level of health.

Staying with our example of intestinal toxins we shall consider the digestive tract of a child, here we see that there are in fact many foods that the child is not able to digest; this is due to the underdevelopment of many related systems; mucous membranes, liver, pancreas etc and because the necessary enzymes have not yet developed, this effectively makes some foods poisonous to that child. These foods together with other toxins may reach crisis levels causing the reactions of vomiting and diarrhoea as noted above.

Now, after the resolution of such an illness the initial presence of some of those new foods may have also been enough to stimulate the production of sufficient digestive enzyme such that the child is now more able to cope with those foods after the illness. This is one mechanism among many that would have developed through the process of that illness.

The important point to note here is that we can observe how the immune system, in conjunction with all the systems of the body, develops through a process of 'learning', as a consequence the individual is less susceptible to the problem after the successful resolution of the illness.

The body is in fact artificially separated into separate systems to enable us to communicate our understanding of them, the digestive system, endocrine system, neurological system, immune system, even the emotional system and so on, however in reality they all operate as one, and the effects of one will involve the other. Learning, thought to be a property of our nervous system and brain, does of course occur with all of our systems.

6.1.2 Resolution of illness with no change in susceptibility.

It is also possible that the result of diarrhoea and vomiting, eliminating toxins in our digestive tract, after for example eating something toxic, has successfully eliminated the toxin but we haven't actually learnt from the process and would be just as likely to react in the same way if we were to eat the same substance again.

6.1.3 Unresolved illness leading to increased susceptibility.

Here, because of one or a combination of our three factors determining the outcome of acute disease (high ingestion of toxins, low vitality and or symptom suppression) we see that the toxic load in the digestive tract was not fully eliminated leaving an unresolved disease. Here it is most significant to realise that the acute symptoms lead to chronic symptoms. The intense nausea, vomiting and diarrhoea in the acute phase result in a less intense but more persistent feeling of nausea and general unease in the chronic phase.

It is highly significant to appreciate that the chronic symptoms result as a failure of the acute symptoms to deal with a particular problem. The acute symptoms are intense and short-lived, with the chronic symptoms being of a similar nature but less intense and long-lived, they can of course persist for much longer than the acute disease perhaps indefinitely.

6.1.4 The illness is not resolved leading to the death of the patient.

Some traumas are so great that the individual does not have the resources to deal with them and cannot recover at all, which leads to the death of the patient; the acute reaction is not sufficient to deal with the problem. Again, notice that the trauma, not the reaction, has lead to the death of the patient, if a patient is sufficiently weak and has accumulated more toxin than they are capable of dealing with, then they could simply die in their attempt to eliminate, when for example producing symptoms of diarrhoea.

There are many under developed countries where mal-nourished children commonly die from diarrhoea and its associated dehydration, this is not because diarrhoea is a killer disease, if it were, then it would be just as likely to kill children in other parts of the world. Clearly it doesn't, and more significantly, symptoms of diarrhoea are important reactions in the resolution of intestinal toxicity. Children that die after symptoms of diarrhoea are suffering from a combination of the factors that influence the outcome of acute disease; high toxic load (toxic stress), low vitality (poor nutritional status) and/or uninformed symptom suppression, which then lead to the secondary complications of dehydration etc.

6.2 "Learning" – a function of mind and body

"The aim of science is not to open the door to infinite wisdom, but to set a limit to infinite error"

Bertolt Brecht

6.2.1 Is sickness a fundamental aspect of the development of individuals?

Acute reactions occur as a result of crisis, in the above example we looked at the build-up of intestinal toxins, the successful resolution of which would ideally lead to the development of the individual. Such development, as distinguished by any learning process, is actually achieved by a process of trial & error and trial & success and this process of learning is in fact common to our whole physical, mental and emotional being.

We can appreciate that there are inherent risks involved with any learning process, the extent and consequence of our error is the price we pay for the benefit of our learning. Ideally, once we understand the nature of our development and the goal of our learning, we are able to determine the best way forward. We clearly need to stimulate learning in significantly small enough steps to minimise the consequences of error, whilst gently allowing the individual to move forward.

Too much stimulation could lead to too much crisis and the consequences of error are too great, therefore the ability to learn diminishes. On the other hand no stimulation, no risk with no possibility of error maintains the status quo, the individual does not move forward; a child forever attached to the mother, unable to independently move, permanently on breast milk.

> *Development is, of course, more than just desirable, it is a biological necessity.*

6.2.2 Learning to digest

Using the example of the digestive tract, in the development of the child to the adult, initially a new-born child will have sensitive and leakier membranes, fewer of the beneficial intestinal microbes, less developed enzymes and digestive juices. In order to develop digestive function the child would need to start on a simple food, such as breast milk and be slowly weaned onto more complex foods.

If too many new complex foods are introduced too quickly then this stress cannot be accommodated and the child would react with vomiting and diarrhoea. Obviously if we persisted adding more and more complex foods this would of course add to the digestive stress creating more symptoms, inhibiting digestion, which would be immediately detrimental to the development of the digestive function of the child.

On the other hand if the child was to be kept on breast milk exclusively for years and years without the introduction of new foods, there would of course be no possibility of overstressing the digestive system but then digestive function would not develop and we would effectively delay physical and emotional development.

Obviously we need to introduce new complex foods to stimulate the development of digestive function in small enough steps to minimise the consequences of possible error, but we cannot of course completely eliminate error without eliminating the introduction of new foods and thereby eliminating the learning process itself.

We can draw similar analogies to any physical, behavioural or emotional learning procedure and realise that the whole mind/body learns and develops as an integrated being and that it is therefore possible to gain insights into the mechanisms of learning by looking at any biological, mental or emotional learning process.

6.2.3 One step forward

If we take for example the process of learning to walk we shall be able to draw relevant analogies to help our understanding. Giving that we have a child about to embark on the process of learning to walk we could agree that the first thing the child needs to learn is how to stand up. Of course we are all aware that the next most likely course of events is that the child will fall.

Much as we would like to be able to learn without making mistakes we actually know that this is not possible, our child will fall. So what we do is minimise the consequences of the fall, learning to walk in a safe environment etc but what we cannot do is eliminate the inherent risk of actually falling. Falling is an intrinsic part of the process; we all know this. So what happens next? Inevitably the child will stand again and eventually learn to balance, take the first step and so on.

It is important to appreciate two essential stages in the learning process; firstly the successful resolution of the problem of falling down is resolved by standing up again, the error of falling has not been so great that the child is unable to try again. However, initially the child will be just as likely to fall again and so we see that although the falling has initially been resolved the susceptibility to falling again is the same. However at some point the resolution of falling by standing is eventually accompanied by balance i.e. a reduced susceptibility to falling down again. It is of course vitally important that balance is accomplished and not simply standing and falling; otherwise we master standing only to be just as susceptible to falling down again. Therefore once we have successfully resolved a problem we are then **less susceptible** to that problem afterwards; this is 'the learning process'. This, by the way, in spite of the major advances in computer technology, remains something that computers and artificial intelligence have not yet been able to achieve.

6.2.4 A grief in your life or a life of grief

Using another example we shall illustrate how emotional development follows similar lines.

The whole progression of childhood development is inextricably linked to the process of separation and other issues of boundaries etc; again we know that this will involve a certain amount of emotional upset. We want to minimise them, but we know they will happen; a child going to school or nursery may experience the trauma of separation from the main carer, usually mother, this experience would be responded to by an expression of grief, i.e. crying. This is again a necessary reaction helping the child to resolve the trauma of separation.

Similarly the experience may be resolved that day, the grief diminishes and all normalises, but this may be followed by a similar expression of grief the following day as the child is taken to school again. As illustrated before, the successful resolution may still not change the susceptibility to that particular trauma straight away. Eventually however something does change, the separation experienced is responded to with tears but the resolution enables the child to deal with subsequent experiences more easily, the child does not cry when being left at school on subsequent days. The child has learnt, there has been a step forward in development and the child is now **less susceptible** to those traumas than before.

But what happens if a grief is not resolved, why would this happen? Firstly, if the trauma was so great that it was not possible for the child to resolve this, given their present capabilities or secondly if their expression of grief was suppressed, if for some reason they felt, or were made to feel, that they could not cry or express their upset, this would be the suppression of the very process that helps them to resolve the emotional trauma.

Suppressing the expression of grief could result in the experience being 'unresolved'. If you force a child to stop crying, as you can well appreciate, the grief does not simply go away, the child may be left feeling sad. The acute grief (intense symptoms with tears, for a relatively short duration) is now replaced by sadness i.e. chronic symptoms (less intense symptoms that can continue for much longer). The child will now be **more susceptible** to that upset after the suppression of their reaction. The grief would not be resolved and they are in fact **sensitised** to those traumas. The mother on retrieving her child may find that the child is more attached than before the experience of school.

From the few examples above we can see that the development of the individual is what is desirable, occasionally events and choices in our lives precipitate in crisis. Ideally development occurs with a minimum of stimulation to avoid real crisis but enough to result in resolution and learning, i.e. resulting in a reduced susceptibility to trauma and an increased ability to live in a greater diversity of conditions. This is effectively what we are craving for when we desire immunity to disease, the ability to withstand the traumas that could result in our disease response.

Immune development in the wider sense involves the ability to deal with our environment independently of our parents. The body has to learn to deal with, complex foods, environmental poisons, heat, cold, humidity, separation, to accommodate diverse microbial populations within the body, develop physical strength, mental ability, and emotional stability etc, any one of those issues in excess would create a stress and promote a symptom reaction leaving the individual ill at-ease, the dis-ease would reflect the amount of stress and would be an expression of our innate susceptibility.

The idea that we can completely eliminate disease by suppressing reactions to disease, (suppressing symptoms) stems from a misinterpretation of the function of symptoms. It is possible to minimise the consequences and the severity of illness by reducing the necessary stimulation in human development, but it is not feasible to eliminate illness unless you completely remove all possibility of development and learning.

CHAPTER 6 - SUMMARY

> Because the body's symptom reactions have an intelligent and vital purpose, those reactions can either succeed or fail in that purpose.

> There are certain factors that determine success or failure, the level of stress/trauma the patient is reacting to, the vitality of the patient and the type of treatment given supportive or suppressive.

> There are also four possible outcomes of an acute disease, the success or failure of the acute reaction can lead to – (1) resolution and learning, (2) resolution and status quo, (3) unresolved and chronic disease or (4) death.

> The ideal objective in overcoming an acute disease would be to resolve the stress/trauma and to have learnt to deal with it in a way that leads to a reduced susceptibility to that issue; i.e. any similar stress experienced in the future is more easily dealt with, it may not appear as a stress, we produce no symptoms of disease, we are more adaptable and have therefore gone through a process of 'learning'.

> Learning occurs in the physical, mental and emotional aspects of our being.

> Diseases are dynamic reactions of the body they are not things and chronic diseases are persistent reactions that continue after the acute reactions have failed to resolve an issue, these reactions continue even if the original stress is no longer there.

> Persisting reactions appearing as chronic disease can also occur if you are under a continual and persistent stress, remove the stress and the chronic disease stops.

CHAPTER SEVEN

7 What happens when the body fails to resolve an illness?

The body has the ability to change strategy when previous attempts at resolving a problem have failed.

7.1 Intestinal toxins

Going back to our central example of intestinal toxicity, remember that in attempting to eliminate toxins from the digestive tract the body is still managing to keep these toxins on the outside membranes of the body, note that only when toxins have crossed the membrane of the digestive tract will they have access to your internal systems and blood supply.

We have established that the build-up of intestinal toxins would be responded to by a reaction of vomiting and diarrhoea, we are also aware of the possible outcomes of the acute reaction, our dis-ease:

> ➢ Resolve and all's well, having learnt from the process we are in fact less susceptible to those issues than before.
> ➢ Resolve but we are just as susceptible; we are effectively waiting for the next crisis and a repeat reaction, unless we can change lifestyle.
> ➢ Unresolve and the toxins remain; we have a chronic disease reaction with mild but sustained nausea and loose stools.

> In rare and severe cases the unresolved illness could lead to the death of the patient.

With unresolved illness, the body could in fact muster up some more energy to react again and we would experience the initial symptoms recurring. However if the build-up of toxins were considered to be a considerable threat, the body would not waste valuable energy in merely repeating a response that had previously failed. There would be a step up in its attempts to detoxify and eliminate the potential poisons and this would therefore lead to an **inflammatory response**.

7.2 Inflammation

The inflammatory response has basically one major purpose and that is to bring immune cells (white blood cells) to an area with high toxicity or damaged cells, with the sole intention of detoxifying, breaking down and eliminating those disease elements.

Inflammation therefore involves the transport of these 'white blood cells' to the specific area of the body once there has been a build-up of sufficient toxicity or an occurrence of considerable injury and tissue damage. This response is at first local, i.e. it involves a specific area of the body as opposed to the whole body and is characterised by the following features.

> Redness – Caused by the widening (dilation) of blood vessels bringing more blood to the area.
> Swelling - Caused by the infiltration of white blood cells into the affected area. This happens because the blood vessel walls and the digestive tract membrane become more permeable (i.e. more porous, the membrane effectively containing more holes) allowing the white blood cells to pass from the blood vessels and out into the GI tract.
> Heat – Caused in part by the increased circulation to the area and partly by the detoxification reactions occurring.

> ➤ Pain – Sometimes due to the physical swelling of the tissue, which is therefore a pointer to help the individual to protect and immobilise that area. Pain is also partly due to the toxins and their effect on the nervous system.

The above therefore characterises a local inflammatory response all of which are vital for the successful detoxification and elimination of poisons that have accumulated in that particular part of the body.

7.2.1 Diagrammatical representation
Inflammation – Blood vessels bringing white blood cells

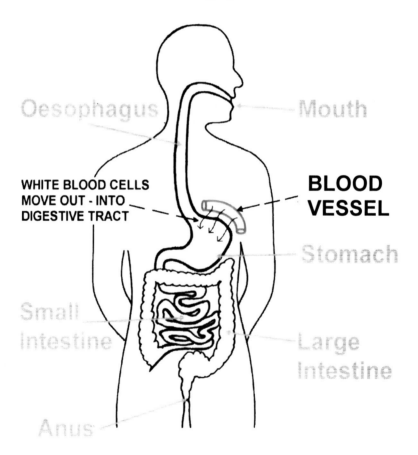

WHITE BLOOD CELLS
MOVE OUT - INTO
DIGESTIVE TRACT

BLOOD VESSEL

Oesophagus

Mouth

Stomach

Small Intestine

Large Intestine

Anus

In the first instance, our inflammatory reactions occur in these 'outside spaces'; ears, nose, throat, digestive tract, lungs, bladder associated outlets and ducts. Therefore with an inflammatory response those additional white blood cells, from the internal blood and lymphatic systems of the body, will have to cross the membrane of the blood vessel and the outer membrane of the body in order to get to the outer spaces of the digestive tract, urinary tract or respiratory tract.

It is in these spaces that toxic build up is likely to occur first, which may also be accompanied by microbe imbalances, some of which however have been demonstrated to have a positive cleaning up effect on dead tissue and toxins, what you may have called an infection. However, in the vast majority of cases, an infection, as such, is not an accurate description of the process of illness, given that the microbes would have been there to start with; we effectively have an accumulation of microbes that have always been present. An accumulation of microbes caused as a direct result of the build-up of toxins, as opposed to an infection of microbes from an external source.

The involvement of white blood cells in the inflammatory response characterises a 'step-up' in the detoxification process, they are able to engulf pathogenic (disease causing) elements and dead tissue, digest and break them down producing broken down waste products ready for their elimination from the body with accompanying phlegm, pus, vomit and diarrhoea. The heat produced is also hostile to certain organisms associated with disease.

7.3 Generalised inflammatory response

This 'local' inflammatory reaction (i.e. in one particular area of the body) could eventually develop into a generalised (whole body) inflammatory response. Here we see symptoms of local heat pain and swelling becoming fever, malaise and general raised white blood cell count. In the 'whole body' response, greater effort is exerted in order to eliminate toxins and address microbial imbalances and the whole body diverts energy away from normal every day activity to immune activity, this kind of diversion of resources or energy is common in human physiology.

Examples of 'Energy Diversion' in biological systems:

There are many examples of activities in human physiology that will decrease to allow other activities to increase.

➢ The classic adrenalin response when fearful, requiring intense muscular activity and a great supply of oxygen to the muscles (during extreme physical activity - running away or fighting for survival) will be accompanied by a coordinated response that decreases digestive function and immune function.

➢ After a heavy meal requiring increased digestive function, blood supply is taken away from the peripheral tissues and muscles and diverted to digestive organs and liver, which may leave the individual feeling tired.

➢ During an intense generalised inflammatory response normal functioning is drastically reduced away from muscular activity and digestion, such that the patient may be barely able to walk and does not want to eat.

7.4 The Benefit of Fever

Symptoms of the generalised inflammatory response are therefore part of a sophisticated and coordinated whole body response that results in symptoms of fever, malaise, tiredness and generalised raised white blood cell count. There is therefore **no** mal-function and once again the symptoms themselves are not the problem but the reaction to the problem.

Reduce the fever – using aspirin, for instance - and the disease may last longer as Timothy Doran of John Hopkins University, Baltimore has demonstrated in the case of chickenpox, published in *Journal of Paediatrics* 114:1045-8 (1989).

The fear that the fever may rise uncontrollably and lead to febrile convulsions is often cited as the justification for the use of fever suppressants (anti-pyretics) and anti-inflammatories. A febrile convulsion can happen when a patient, often a child, has a high fever and they become almost comatose, limp and apparently lifeless with initial and occasional twitching. The term convulsion can give the impression that the symptoms are mainly convulsive, spasmodic and epileptic in nature; however a febrile convulsion is not a neurological fit, the main state is one of limpness and lifelessness. Here the body has in fact diverted almost all its resources to raising a fever, dealing with the diseased tissue and toxicity. Once again, even in the case of a febrile convulsion, the symptoms are in fact part of a coordinated response to the trauma.

The fear is that the fever will destroy cellular components of the body and the febrile convulsion will lead to permanent neurological damage. However studies do in fact show the opposite, that fevers and febrile convulsions cause no damage. So the use of this rationale to sell drugs must have either originated in belief from fear or simply used as pharmaceutical sales leverage.

When the body produces a fever the temperature regulation is **not** out of control, but the thermostat has simply been set to a higher level to deal with the trauma. In fact there are internal mechanisms within the body to stop the fever running above a certain temperature. From standard medical texts there has been no evidence of cellular damage caused by fever, and in fact it seems hard to believe that the body would simply cook itself. The sporadic very high rises in temperature (spiking) that occur whilst a patient develops a fever, would be more likely to occur if they are taking fever suppressants, because as the drug is naturally metabolised by the body and therefore wears off, the fever spikes to higher than natural levels as the body counteracts the original suppression.

Rather than the fever causing long-term neurological damage, it is the internal toxins and concomitant microbes, if not eliminated, that will damage the internal systems including the nervous system. Therefore suppressing the fever to avoid neurological damage is actually doing the exact opposite, pre-disposing the patient to invasive toxicity and the very symptoms that one is trying to avoid.

The term *'Fever Phobia'* was used by Barton Schmitt, MD, back in 1980 to describe the numerous misconceptions that many parents and health professionals (including doctors) had, about fever. Twenty years later as reported in the journal 'Paediatrics' a similar study demonstrated that fever phobia still exists and recommends further studies to evaluate how to re-educate the public and health professionals.

An alternative view one might think...the following comment from Wouter H Havinga, General practitioner appeared in the British Medical Journal 314. 7th June 1997 page 1692:

> *"... The common understanding of the general public seems to be that when fever gets too high it can cause death. In hospitals this seems to be confirmed, because paracetamol is given whenever a patient has a fever. I have not, however, seen a publication to support this. This misunderstanding has major implications for general practice. A paper by Kai illustrates this.*
>
> *Current understanding is that people die of the underlying illness, not of fever. To support the benefit of fever one can start with the evolutionary argument. If fever were not of value for survival it would not be part of our defence.*
>
> *Research has shown that many immune responses are enhanced by an increase in temperature. Routine antipyretic treatment for fever is generally unnecessary and conceivably harmful. It has been suggested that it may prolong illness and increase or prolong viral shedding.*

Parents do not need to worry about febrile convulsions, because when they telephone for advice the fever is already established and the episode of a rapid rise in temperature will have passed. Febrile convulsions, understandably, distress parents, but parents can be reassured that convulsions will not cause a disability. Also, the outcome is determined more by the underlying cause than by the seizures themselves.

In conclusion, and in line with the views of Styrt and Sugerman, I would like to see routine antipyretic treatment reassessed and adjusted, depending on whether desired objectives such as, reduction of cardiovascular stress and increase in comfort are being achieved.

I think that paracetamol should be taken off the market.... *If this were done to coincide with a national campaign explaining the benefits of fever then it would have a major educational effect on the general public. Consequently, this would reduce the number of consultations and would probably enhance the health of the nation.*

The role of fever as adaptive and immune enhancing appears to be acknowledged in conventional medical circles, it has also been found that death rates increase in patients who are less able to produce a sufficiently high fever in response to infections (American Journal of Medicine. 68:344-355, 1980 - Bernard E. Kreger, Donald E. Craven, William R. McCabe). The extensive use of anti-pyretics would therefore appear to be as a result of very effective pharmaceutical sales, as opposed to clinical evidence.

Going back to our example of toxic build up within the digestive tract; this would give rise to a local inflammation (e.g. a gastritis), leading to a generalised inflammatory response with fever; if the body has been successful in eliminating toxins and redressing microbial imbalances, then recovery takes place and normal functioning resumes. However, from an orthodox pharmaceutical perspective if we perceive the inflammation as being the problem itself we are apt to treat the body by giving **anti-inflammatory** medication and therefore make it more difficult for the body to deal with the underlying cause, and if unsuccessful in our attempts to deal with those causes using inflammatory reactions, we find our pathology takes on a significantly new dimension.

CHAPTER 7 - SUMMARY

> The type of symptom reactions of the body will change to adopt a new strategy of healing if the current reactions are failing.

> The body will divert energy away from different activities towards immune functions when under significant immune stress.

> Inflammation is the coordination and mobilisation of immune cells and chemicals to an area of dead tissue or toxins.

> Fever is part of the inflammatory healing reaction, suppressing the fever will make it harder to succeed in resolving the immune challenge.

CHAPTER EIGHT

8 Breaking through the outer barrier and into the body

If these new strategies fail, then the body's external defences are breached and our illness enters a significantly new phase,

Up until this point in our story; toxins, microbes and symptom reactions, have been kept on the external parts of the body, (remember outside of the body means external to the outer skin and inner mucous membranes of the digestive tract, lungs, urinary tract). This next phase involves crossing over to the inner systems of the body, blood, lymph, organs and nerves.

With our situation unresolved, i.e. the symptoms have been unable to eliminate toxins from the digestive tract, then, persistent toxins can leak across the membrane into the blood supply and internal tissues. This therefore poses a more serious threat to the normal functioning of your body.

It is also possible that toxins normally excreted from the blood accumulate in the blood as elimination is now compromised. Up to this point, toxins have been maintained in our external spaces, from an immune and therefore protective point of view this is one of the significant purposes of the immune system, to eliminate waste products and keep toxins out of our internal systems beyond the barrier of the respiratory, urinary and digestive membranes as well as the external skin.

8.1 Across the membrane into the blood

However, once toxins do start to accumulate in the blood, then a whole new array of immune elements comes into play. As the situation deteriorates with toxins leaking back across the membranes of our eliminatory systems (going from outside to inside) entering the blood supply, microbial elements may also traverse with them.

We need to remind ourselves that there are many microbes normally present on these outer membranes that have their various functions as described previously and if these outer membranes break down then microbes as well as toxins may now enter your blood. Initially the smaller microbes will leak across the membranes first; therefore viruses will cross far more readily than the larger bacteria cells, (viruses being much smaller than bacteria). We also know that your cells will produce viruses when poisoned, and therefore viruses can accumulate internally as a result of blood poisoning.

Viral illnesses, such as; measles, rubella and chicken pox, culminating in the typical viral rash, is the end result of the elimination of toxins and cell debris across the membranes of the body including the skin. The viral particles are just one of the components of cell debris. As such theses viral illnesses are indicative of milder blood toxicity and less membrane permeability than that of bacterial septicaemia, wherein bacteria, which are much larger than viruses have managed to traverse the outer membranes of the body.

Remember also that viruses are thought to be pathogenic (disease causing) when they infect cells and hijack the cellular building machinery to make more viruses. We must remember that this is a theory that we have been unable to confirm using the modern techniques of electron microscopy. Evidence so far also suggests that viral particles, if at all present, can be caused by cell breakdown and therefore viruses are the consequence of disease due to cellular poisoning.

Toxins, by their nature, are called toxins because of the effects they have on your cells, when such toxins enter the blood system they may infect and affect cells, causing cellular destruction or malfunction producing cell debris including viral particles. As a consequence, the internal blood leukocytes (white blood cells) can recognise these damaged cells, destroying them and preparing them for elimination. These leukocytes are specialised immune cells operating in the blood system and they come into play once sufficient toxins and damage has occurred beyond the membranes of the body into the blood system and internal organs. The activity of these white blood cells (leukocytes) in acute blood toxicity will be a part of a generalised inflammatory response and will be accompanied by fever, malaise, loss of appetite, etc.

8.2 The antibody in real life

B-cells are specific white blood cells that produce antibodies (antibodies are long chain protein molecules) and these antibodies are able to attach to foreign elements within the blood, in classical immunology this attachment is often described as a lock and key mechanism. The foreign element (the key) attracts an antibody (the lock) that is able to wrap around a portion of the foreign object (the part that the antibody binds to is called the antigen) this newly shaped antibody then instructs other B cells to produce exact copies of these antibodies so that they can quickly attach to other similar foreign elements getting in the blood.

A simple and true story may help to focus our understanding on the issues here; a father, tired of his children continually leaving their pet dog poo in the garden, decides to put flags around the garden indicating the places where they need to clean up. Like antibodies theses flags guide where the clean-up operation needs to occur, but they do no cleaning themselves and the more efficient the clean-up operation the less flags we see. This is why we find people that are immune to illnesses and yet have no antibodies for the microbes that are classically associated with those illnesses.

So we see that antibodies themselves are **not** able to carry out the function of detoxification, breakdown and elimination, antibodies seem to function by identifying certain components, flagging them and enabling the other leukocytes (immune cells) to notice them, it is these other immune cells that detoxify and eliminate the flagged foreign elements from the body.

However it is also worth noting that many kinds of white blood cells do not need these antibodies in order to carry out efficient immune clean-up, it has been demonstrated that successful immune responses involving these leukocytes (granulocytes, macrophages and other immune cells such as natural killer cells) are able to detoxify and eliminate toxins and damaged cells without the formation of antibodies.

Prior to the work of immunologist Dr. Merrill W. Chase in 1940's, scientists believed that the body mounted its attacks against pathogens primarily through <u>antibodies</u> circulating in the blood stream, known as humoral immunity.

The research of Dr Chase on white blood cells helped undermine the longstanding belief that antibodies alone protected the body from disease and micro-organisms, Dr. Chase made his landmark discovery in the early 1940's while working with Dr. Karl Landsteiner, a Nobel laureate recognized for his work identifying the human blood groups.

> **"This was a major discovery because everyone now thinks of the immune response in two parts...in many instances it's the cellular components that are more important than antibodies,"**

Dr. Michel Nussenzweig, professor of immunology at Rockefeller.

Many leukocytes are capable of recognition, learning and memory, many of which do not need antibodies to function in destruction and elimination of toxins, viruses and affected cells. This is one reason why one can perform efficient immune activity without the production of antibodies.

Antibody stimulation involved in allergies and asthma

Antibodies are produced by specialised immune cells called 'B-Cells' and there is evidence to suggest that individuals with poor immune function seem to produce a high B-cell/antibody responses and low cellular responses. The New England Journal of Medicine, (Jan 30, 1992; 326: 298-304) reports that people with allergies, asthma, and diseases of an autoimmune origin show this bias towards antibody production.

Mario Clerci of the National Cancer Institute in the US suggests for example, that by looking at HIV positive patients i.e. the ones that are producing antibodies, we're looking at the immune failures.

8.2.1 Autoimmune disease related to B cells and antibodies

It was generally thought that autoimmune diseases, where the body appears to be attacking itself, was a misguided immune assault on our own cells brought about by a mal-function or misrecognition by the active T-cells. However it is now increasingly apparent from recent research that anti-bodies to our own cellular components are produced before symptoms appear, as discovered in Lupus and Type 1 diabetes. We know that vaccines have been shown to contribute to both of these conditions and now there are therapeutic approaches to dampen the activity of B-cells, the immune cells involved in antibody production.

Nature Reviews Drug Discovery, 5, 564-576 (July 2006)

So it appears we are going full circle creating more and more vaccines to stimulate the immune system to produce anti-bodies via B-cell stimulation and now with the formation of autoimmune disorders researchers are desperately trying to dampen down the B-cell responses.

So the pre-occupation of vaccine promoters in trying to stimulate B-cells in the blood to produce high antibody responses without any regard to cellular immune function, is based on a pre-1940 theory of immunology that has since been proved wrong. It is likely that the £billion vaccine industry is entirely misguided and has yet to acknowledge what we have known about the immune system for some time. Over stimulating one arm of the immune system with vaccines creates illnesses that require a compensatory dampening using yet more pharmaceutical intervention.

Do vaccinators know what they are doing with the intricately balanced components of the human immune system?

8.3 The Rash

As a result of this generalised inflammatory response and blood immune activity by the white blood cells; destruction and elimination of blood toxins, cell debris and microbes, then the resolution of this internal blood toxicity would lead to the successful elimination of toxins and cell debris (viruses).

Elimination out of the blood, back across the membranes of the body to the outside, often results in a skin **rash**. The rash is in fact the visible process of elimination through the skin; because the blood has access to the external skin, as well as the external environments provided by the membranes of the lungs, urinary and digestive tracts, any part of this skin and membrane system can be the site used to eliminate toxins and cell debris. Once again, symptoms of phlegm, coughing, sneezing, nasal discharge, and less occasionally vomiting and diarrhoea may accompany the rash.

The rash, even within an orthodox context is known to be a vital component of the immune response and is termed viral shedding. The Lancet Jan 5th 1985 reports on an orthodox study conducted in Holland, investigating the phenomenon of measles virus infection **without** the appearance of typical measles rash.

In the patients studied, for those with antibodies but NO history of measles rash by adulthood, (average age in the study was 38 years), there was shown to be an increased incidence of immunoreactive diseases, sebaceous skin diseases, degenerative diseases of bone and cartilage, and certain tumours.

The report concludes that, at the time of infection, it may be dangerous to interfere with the immune response by administering a passive immunisation to suppress the rash. It also states...

> *"The absence of a rash may imply that intracellular virus (poisons) escapes neutralisation during the acute infection and this, in turn, might give rise to the development of diseases subsequently".*
>
> **The Lancet, 5 January 1985 (325; 8419; 1 – 5)**

The rash would therefore appear to be vitally important, indeed with regard to the rest of the blood immune response the Lancet report goes on to state that further studies in children with agammaglobulinaemia i.e. **children unable to produce antibodies**, find that they are able to produce a rash, overcome the illness and develop immunity just as other children. Whereas those with impaired cellular immunity (unable to produce sufficient leukocyte responses) are more likely to develop complications such as pneumonia and possibly die.

It is interesting to note in homeopathy and naturopathy that not only is the rash an important symptom in the resolution of blood toxicity illnesses, such as measles, but also of equal importance is the pattern of the appearance and disappearance of the rash, i.e. the direction of the movement of the rash. Essentially, 'if' the symptoms are curative leading to resolution, then the rash starts higher up the body and moves its way down, finally disappearing from the lowest parts of the legs. It has similarly been documented in homeopathic literature that if in fact the rash moves from down to up, the opposite way, then the illness is not resolving and could therefore lead to more internal problems (or if fortunate, a recurrence of the rash).

The appearance of the rash in this generalised inflammatory response is caused by the blood vessels at the surface of the skin dilating at points causing the red spots, and the membrane of the blood vessels and skin, becoming more permeable (more leaky) allowing toxins and viruses out. The red blood cells and most other blood components are still confined to the blood vessels; only toxins, viruses and the flexible white blood cells can get out.

Note this is distinctly different from the severe toxaemia found in cases of septicaemia, where there is extreme blood toxicity often involving the presence of bacteria. At the site of the rash the blood vessel walls break down and there is blood loss under the surface of the skin giving the appearance of the septicaemic rash. This is not an eliminatory rash; the patient is effectively bleeding under the skin as a result of extreme poisoning, the blood is not contained within the blood vessels, it is a non-blanching rash and therefore the classic test of pressing a glass on the skin shows that the rash does not disappear. Generalised septicaemia can only happen under conditions of extreme blood poisoning and severe immune breakdown, once you understand the pattern and purpose of disease symptoms it is possible to predict the circumstances that lead to this scenario and it can therefore be effectively avoided.

The resolution of blood toxicity as described in the generalised inflammatory reaction in for example measles, results in the successful **elimination** of the toxins from the blood and internal systems. Remember that in our example of toxicity in the digestive tract, the build-up of toxins enabled some to leak into the blood system across the stomach membrane. During the curative inflammatory response that followed there would have been:

> ➢ An increase in permeability in both the **blood vessel walls** and the **membranes of the digestive tract**, (more porous, with larger spaces/holes) to allow an active elimination of white blood cells, toxins and microbes back out across the membranes of the digestive tract.

> ➤ During this time there would have been a decrease in appetite and digestive function, so that food elements and other toxins are not able to pass across the membrane to the blood whilst the body is eliminating toxins in the opposite direction back across the membrane from the blood.

It is significant to realise that after the successful elimination of these toxins, cell debris and microbes, normal function resumes and as such **the membranes reduce their permeability once again**, i.e. the spaces within the membranes, that have previously allowed the toxins and white blood cells to travel out, reduce back to normal.

Therefore it is also possible to see how the membrane adapts and as with all of our learning processes, we know that **if there is resolution and learning** culminating in a reduced susceptibility to disease, then the individual (and therefore the biological system) is effectively stronger. If the individual has not resolved the illness then they will be left with chronic symptoms (persistent low level symptoms) and will be weaker i.e. be more susceptible to disease.

It therefore follows that the membrane itself, rather than just going back to normal (as it was before) actually becomes stronger after a **successful** immune response. The individual would in fact be far less susceptible to toxins entering the system; consequently 'immunity' as such, is much more general and corresponds to the resistance to a whole host of toxins and associated viral elements entering the body.

However, if the response has been **unsuccessful** - culminating in chronic disease - the membrane does not go back to normal, but in fact **remains slightly permeable**, thus persistently allowing small amounts of toxins in, and in fact the individual is left more susceptible to disease.

To summarise:

In order to successfully produce an eliminatory skin rash the body needs to have experienced a build-up of toxins internally within the blood, which are broken down and engulfed by white blood cells, resulting in the process of elimination through the skin, culminating in the rash.

This is a process that needs to be learnt and as such is part of the immune development of the individual which normally occurs during childhood.

8.4 Childhood development in relation to immune function

At birth children do not have a fully functional immune system, for example they are unable to produce a generalised inflammatory response with fever until a period of time after birth, and this has been estimated as taking three months but of course depends on the individual.

The membranes of the digestive, urinary, respiratory tracts and skin are more permeable than in adulthood, allowing in more potential poisons. The main detoxification organ, the liver, has not developed the necessary enzymes and metabolic processes that enable one to detoxify toxins. The Lymphatic system and therefore T-cells and B-cells are similarly under developed, along with other immune cells.

It is estimated that 80% of the immune function is in the digestive system; in fact there is considerable overlap between immune function and digestive function. Enzymes are capable of breaking down both toxins and large food substances to smaller easily absorbed molecules, with the digestive tract membrane having the ability to keep out toxins and larger food substances but able to selectively absorb smaller nutrients.

In our example of blood toxicity; with the successful elimination of blood toxins and microbes in a child (the first illnesses of childhood, measles, rubella, chickenpox etc) the body has learnt an immune process that it has not been able to do before. The immune cells have developed memory and the membranes themselves have become stronger and less porous. The role of the membranes has often been undervalued in the portrayal of immunity and yet they provide the first lines of defence to our external environment.

Classically 'immune memory' was attributed to the presence of antibodies, however we now know that antibodies are not always present after successful immune reactions, we also know that other leukocytes have memory capabilities, the membrane itself with hormone receptor sites, selective channels and selective absorption also has memory. It is likely, given the nature of the human body and immune function that almost every element has memory and learning capability.

What happens if the body isn't able to eliminate toxins via the skin and therefore unable to produce a rash, or if in fact the rash doesn't fully resolve the internal toxicity?

8.5 Unresolved Blood Toxicity

The significance of immunity as a learning process shall become even more apparent when we consider the consequences of failed immune responses. If the elimination of blood toxins, cell debris and viral particles has been unsuccessful, you would have a condition akin to a 'post-viral syndrome'. A syndrome where the problem of blood toxicity has been unresolved, i.e. the toxins, cell debris and viral particles remain within the blood system. From what we know of immune learning and **unresolved** issues, we know that you become **more** susceptible and therefore sensitised to a problem, if resolution has been unsuccessful.

Reminding ourselves of the consequences of **unresolved** acute disease, we are aware that the intense and short-lived symptoms of acute illness leads to less intense but more persistent symptoms of the chronic illness, we can therefore predict the symptom scenario that an unresolved acute will lead to. An unresolved acute inflammatory reaction would lead to persisting symptoms of low-intensity inflammation in the system.

> ➢ The acute symptoms; increased blood supply to the membranes, increased permeability in both the blood vessel walls and the membranes of the digestive tract, (more porous, with larger spaces/holes), accompanied by a decrease in - appetite, digestive function, and physical function.

> ➢ If chronic we see persistent low intensity acute symptoms; an inability to maintain body temperature, a lack of vital heat - feeling chilly, low physical energy levels, poor appetite and persistently leaky membranes of the digestive tract.

Significantly, with unresolved blood toxicity the membrane is persistently 'leaky', you are now more susceptible to toxins entering your system, in addition to still having the initial internal toxins that have not been eliminated, and you are now **sensitised** to those toxins, **not immune** to them.

Persistent membrane permeability of the digestive tract would allow more toxins into the blood system and in fact certain food elements would gain access to the blood, before they have been fully broken down. These would overburden the detoxifying capacity of the liver and present an immune challenge in the blood. These food elements and toxins would overload immune cell activity in the blood and eventually as more elements enter the blood system, the failure of the cellular response to keep up would lead to the production of antibodies to these particles, as they try to alert the clean-up cells to eliminate these toxic elements.

With persistent membrane permeability we are now starting to develop food sensitivities and as we produce antibodies to our food, we see the development of food allergies. There will be a persisting low level elimination of internal toxins onto the outer membranes of the skin and lungs and we therefore see food sensitivities expressed as chronic skin reactions and chronic lung conditions.

This can also be perceived from the perspective of observable acute symptoms becoming chronic; therefore in the case of an unresolved acute rash this could then lead to a persistent (chronic) rash for example leading to eczema. In this state you are not able to eliminate using an acute (quick and intense) eliminative rash, i.e. you are unable to have measles not as a result of good health but due to poor health.

If the symptoms of eczema (the chronic rash) are further suppressed using, for example a topical steroid, (which is designed to suppress the immune functions of the body), this may offer relief, but does not address the cause of the problem and in fact often leads to a deeper chronic, which we know often leads to asthma, i.e. affecting the lung skin which is considered to be a deeper skin.

CHAPTER 8 – SUMMARY

> The body does it's best to eliminate waste products and keep toxins out of our internal systems beyond the barrier of the respiratory, urinary and digestive membranes as well as the external skin

> If the membranes of the body allow toxins and microbes to enter then a blood immune response initiates, wherein immune cells digest and eliminate unwanted debris and toxins.

> Antibodies can be used to flag up unwanted components in the blood but many immune cells can operate without them which is why immunity can be demonstrated in people with no antibodies.

> In a crisis of blood toxicity eliminating those toxins produces a skin rash, in orthodox medicine this is also known as viral shedding, at the site of the rash the blood vessels are widening creating the red appearance together with the leaking out of toxins through the skin.

> The production of such a rash, for example measles, is a learnt process, if it does not complete fully the symptoms can persist leading to a continuous low level inflammation such as eczema.

> The membranes of the body could then persistently leak, increasing sensitivity to environmental toxins and food.

CHAPTER NINE

9 What's the body up to when creating allergic reactions?

If toxins have crossed the membranes of the body and have failed to be eliminated then the individual becomes sensitised to those substances and then has to develop new strategies to prevent any more of those substances entering the body and causing further problems.

9.1 Allergies

Allergies are often thought of as an 'over-sensitivity' to potentially harmless substances. From an orthodox perspective therefore, we have another example of how the reactions of the body are perceived as 'malfunctions'.

When presenting with such a condition we are told that we have an 'over-reactive' immune system, responding to harmless elements that we need not react to, therefore a condition that we need medication to suppress.

9.2 Is pollen dangerous

We may at first sight presume that surely a substance such as pollen is not dangerous, but these so-called harmless substances that cause immune reactions (substances that are therefore called 'allergens') **are** however potentially harmful if present in the blood. The question as to whether a substance is harmful or not needs to be reframed; we need to specifically ask **where** in the human body, is this substance harmful?

Many food substances, environmental elements, bacteria and viruses are well tolerated within certain spaces of the human body, i.e. in the digestive, genitourinary, respiratory tracts etc., however, place them in your blood, give them access to your internal organs, your cells, enzymes, receptors and nervous system and you have a potentially dangerous situation.

The problem with individuals that have allergies is that they have been exposed to these elements **in their blood**, elements that have therefore managed to cross their immune barriers. This only becomes a problem if they have then not been able to eliminate these elements successfully and they are therefore **sensitised** to them. It has been suggested that the main source of allergens is in fact from the food we eat and that often we react to the last straw that breaks the camel's back, after we have become significantly overloaded with allergens. It is also known as the rain barrel effect, we are able to tolerate a certain amount of blood toxicity until the barrel becomes overloaded and we start to produce symptoms of disease. The proof of this can be seen when individuals are able to exclude the major food allergens that they are sensitive to; they then find that they are much less sensitive to other allergens.

9.3 Allergies - intelligent biological response

However, once the body has become overloaded, it reacts, in an ingenious way, by producing a specific kind of marker. This marker is the antibody IgE, and is a different kind of antibody to the ones that are produced in the blood for example IgM or IgG, (IgG and M, for when we are actively flagging elements that are to be eliminated by other white blood cells).

This IgE is able to recognise those elements that we are sensitised to, i.e. those elements that we are internally overloaded with, that we couldn't eliminate. We position these special antibodies in the places of the body that are most likely to come in contact with these elements first; the membranes of the upper respiratory tract and upper digestive tract, nose, throat, mouth and outer skin etc. The body is then instructed to react to these allergens strongly as soon as we come in contact with them, reactions involving white blood cells and mucus, such as sneezing, coughs, tears, nasal discharges, swelling, etc.

This reaction occurs to these specific elements because your body knows that you have been unable to eliminate these particles and that they will continue to cross your membranes causing problems to your internal systems if you do not stop them from entering your various bodily tracts. The allergic response is a highly intelligent method of alerting you to a problem whilst also creating a mucus and white cell barrier to that substance.

However, once again the pharmaceutical approach to an allergic reaction is to interpret the response as an over-reaction to a harmless substance, once more assuming that the body is mal-functioning and therefore prescribes antihistamines, which are chemicals that block your histamine responses. Histamine is a natural chemical that coordinates the allergic response, attracting white blood cells, dilating blood vessels etc but using an antihistamine, rather than deal with the problem of unresolved toxicity the body is effectively suppressed and therefore stopped from being able to perform its intelligent warning and damage limitation reaction.

This of course has the effect of allowing those substances into the body adding to the toxic load; initially the patient may have repeated allergic reactions, often each new phase of reactions are more severe than the last, such that more and more powerful pharmaceutical drugs have to be given each time. Eventually the allergic reaction itself can become so pronounced that it becomes problematic with the increased swelling in the upper respiratory tract capable of blocking the airways and ultimately threatening the life of the patient.

If however the body is effectively suppressed then the allergic symptoms stop but we find toxins are given more access to the internal systems and we develop deeper and more chronic disease. By looking at illnesses as isolated events in a patient's life and by looking at parts of the body as disconnected to the human whole, the significance of symptom reactions is lost and consequently the dangers of pharmaceutical intervention underestimated.

However in the attempt to join the dots of consequence beyond the freeze frame of individual diseases it has recently been demonstrated by orthodox medical scientists that individuals with allergies are in fact protected from more severe and chronic diseases.

Just as we can demonstrate the benefit of conditions such as measles, mumps and rubella in preventing allergies Nancy Vokers. has reported in the Journal of the National Cancer Institute (J of NCI 1999; 91; 1916-18) that allergy sufferers are less likely to develop cancer.

> *"An overview by the National Cancer Institute reports that allergy sufferers had a 40 percent decreased risk for pancreatic cancer. Even more impressive, research from China, looking at more than 17,000 people, found those who had allergies had 60 percent less of any kind of cancer than those who didn't have allergies.*

> *"And HIV patients who get hay fever have a 65 percent reduced risk of getting non-Hodgkin's lymphoma compared to non-allergic HIV patients. Even the number of bee or wasp stings seemed to reduce the risk and be*

protective against non-Hodgkin's lymphoma, as well." as has been demonstrated.

So there is a correlation between the ability to maintain an allergic reaction and the avoidance of even more severe immune deficient reactions and cancer.

> *"... most of the studies have shown a reduced risk for cancer among people who have a history of allergies. One perspective is that allergies are evidence of the competence of immune system function."*

If we look at this from the point of view of the body trying to limit the effect of poisons in the system: If the **allergic reaction** has been **unsuccessful**, or successfully suppressed, then poisons are given access to the internal systems, and we can therefore see a pattern of disease with regard to the next likely places in the body that will be affected.

Interestingly the same article reports on a study that shows treating the allergy with steroids increases the risk of cancer, which would highlight the possible dangers of suppression again.

> *We saw a reduced risk for [asthmatics] who used bronchodilators alone, no reduced risk for those on bronchodilators and steroids, and an increased risk for those on steroids alone."*

9.4 Desensitisation

The principle of desensitisation is an interesting concept, but depending on the nature of the procedure this may be just as harmful as symptom suppression. Some desensitisation techniques may involve repeated exposure of the allergen to the system so that ultimately the body gives up reacting. This, of course, does not deal with the issue of susceptibility; there is no 'immune learning', but there is in fact 'immune shut-down', wherein the body, as with suppression, eventually gives-up reacting in that particular manner. If there is a problem of blood toxicity and membrane permeability, this is not addressed and once again blood toxins may build-up internally unrestrained by the immune system.

CHAPTER 9 - SUMMARY

> An allergy to something indicates that, the particular substance has previously gained access to the blood (the internal parts of the body) and we have been unable to eliminate it sufficiently.
> Allergic reactions are designed to keep those things away from the body to stop them building up further.
> Allergic substances are harmless on the outside of the body but dangerous if in the blood.
> Allergic reactions become more dangerous the more we suppress them.

CHAPTER TEN

10 The health and disease map

How health deteriorates in stages and why if inappropriately treated, illnesses can become more chronic and more dangerous

10.1 Disease progression

This is a summary of the concept that symptoms have specific functions that can succeed or fail. If these symptom reactions fail they can persist i.e. become chronic and the problem goes deeper into the body.

If these reactions fail to deal with these deeper problems then there are more strategies available, but there is greater potential for damage and if symptoms are suppressed at this stage there is a higher probability of creating more serious consequences.

By understanding the purpose of disease symptoms i.e. the reactions of the body to trauma, we are able to see the consequences of immune success or immune failure. We have been able to show that as a result of immune failure, symptoms persist at a lower intensity and the trauma/problem goes deeper within the system. To add to our predicament we are often given suppressive medication during our acute reactions, which makes it more likely that our reactions will fail.

As such it is possible to plot the progression of acute disease to chronic disease.

This effect is sometimes harder to appreciate in orthodox medicine; **note** that we are not simply looking at the effect of a poison in the system but also the effect of our **failure** to deal with the poison, resulting in **a persistent reaction**.

If we look an extreme example of Post-Traumatic Stress (PTS), imagine an individual in a hostage scenario who is threatened to be killed, he lives in fear of meeting an imminent and violent death. The psychological stress is so great that the mind and body cannot resolve the trauma, so feelings of fear and anxiety persistent at a lower level than might appear appropriate given the gravity of the situation. If it transpires that the hostage is later freed, from this point, greater reactions to the trauma start to manifest; fears, anxiety, flash-backs, dreams, sleeplessness, physical symptoms of anxiety etc.

Even though the source of the trauma has been removed, the patient continues to react as if the trauma was still there. This is exactly the same with the symptoms of the physical body, after a failure to deal with blood poisons through an eliminative rash then a persistent response remains. Even though the poisons may be eventually removed, the immune system remains persistently skewed towards antibody responses, stuck in membrane permeability and therefore more open to invasive toxins, leading to chronic skin reactions, e.g. eczema. and and allergic responses to particular toxins/allergens.

Most orthodox interpretations of disease, as sponsored by the pharmaceutical industry, look at a snap-shot of disease, like a single frame of a movie, the nature of such scientific endeavour then entails a detailed search of the material components of the individual frame. The significance of the symptom response is lost, and the connections to the problems of the past and to the future goals are never integrated, nor the significance of the individual part to the whole. This approach fails to appreciate the 'meaning' of symptoms other than being a measure of deviation from an idealised 'norm'.

10.2 Disease as a 'process' not a 'thing'

By observing the movie as well as the details of each frame, the significance is thrown into light. The reason that membrane permeability exists in chronic disease is because the acute elimination requiring such membrane permeability failed, thus in the chronic disease a low level permeability persists. The reason the immune response is skewed to antibodies instead of the cellular response is because the acute response to poisons involving antibodies as a last resort fails thus the antibody response persists...and so on and so on.

10.3 More 'invasive' consequences

If a patient no longer has the ability to create acute rashes to eliminate blood poisons, and no longer has the ability to stop further entry of toxins with allergic reactions, then the body has to be able to neutralise internal poisons and keep them out of harm's way. Many of these toxins may already be flagged up by antibodies forming persistent immune complexes.

The accumulated immune complexes and other toxins in the internal tissues of the body will be stored in the connective tissue, fat deposits and the joints where they can do the least damage. They will also be found in the lymphatic tissue and in the liver where the body attempts most of the detoxification reactions. By default they may collect in the blood system occasionally at the heart valves and also in the kidneys, where there are very fine capillaries. Consequently these are the most common places where acute and chronic immune reactions occur. Here we see acute and chronic symptoms of cellulitis, arthritis, nephritis, hepatitis, rheumatic heart disease etc.

The body has been doing its best to eliminate toxins, microbes and cellular debris from its interior thereby protecting the internal tissues of the body and it is of course especially important to protect the cells of the **nervous system**.

But when poisons, waste, cell debris and microbes build around the nerve cells, the failure of acute and chronic responses here could lead to severe consequences in terms of acute and chronic neurological damage, resulting in paralysis, loss of sensory function, brain damage and even death. In the acute we see illnesses such as acute flaccid paralysis and infantile paralysis (*later called paralytic poliomyelitis in an attempt to attribute the pathology to the polio virus*), meningitis, encephalitis, and in the chronic, illnesses such as autism, attention deficiency syndromes, ME, Alzheimer's and so on. These are the invasive illnesses that the body is doing its utmost to avoid, but in fact most suppressive medication actually predisposes us to.

A summary of immune events show how the responses of the body become more internalised as the systems become overwhelmed and/or suppressed. Illnesses of the internal systems such as polio, meningitis and encephalitis are not caught but are developed as a result of immune failure. The microbes associated with these illnesses are in everyone and clearly do no harm as they are present naturally on the external membranes of the body.

Illness progression table

OUTSIDE

1 Eliminatory Functions	2 Increased Physical Elimination	3 Inflammatory Response - Local	4 Inflammatory Response - General
• Perspiration • Respiration • Defecation • Urination	• Increased sweat, odour, concentration • Increased respiratory mucus, cough, sneeze, nasal discharge • Vomiting and diarrhoea • Increased concentration & odour of urine	FIRST LOCAL • Redness • Swelling • Heat • Pain • Change of function Blood vessels **DILATE** and there is an increase in membrane **PERMEABILITY**	If not resolved at local place becomes a **GENERAL REACTION** • Fever • Raised white cell count generally • General malaise • Change of general function
NO SYMPTOMS **NO DISCOMFORT** **NO PAIN.**	**FIRST SIGNS OF SYMPTOMS,** MILD DISCOMFORT OR PAIN Build up of mucus and toxins can lead to increase microbes (germs)	**Inflammation** brings white blood cells to an area of dead tissue or toxins. **Microbes** (germs) may increase as a **RESULT of toxicity,** but can also HELP to clean up.	High Immune function. **Forced to physically rest**: Energy diverted from normal function to general immune activity.

INSIDE Across the membrane - Deeper into the body ➔

5 Crossed Outside to Inside	6 Chronic Blood Toxicity	7 Internal organs affected	8 Nervous system affected
GENERALISED INFLAMMATORY REACTION OF THE BLOOD. White blood cells of internal blood & lymph system locate and digest toxins and dead tissue. Elimination of blood toxins resulting in a **SKIN RASH**.	Chronic blood toxicity and **chronic membrane permeability** leads to chronic elimination; eczema, asthma, hayfever, etc. **ALLERGIES:** Damage limitation reactions.	Detoxification of toxins attempted by **liver & lymphatics**. Excess toxins stored in **joints, fat &** connective tissue BUT may adversely affect **kidneys &** blood vessels including **heart/valve**.	Poisoning of brain, spinal cord and peripheral nerves. Leading to: **<u>ACUTE</u>** **Meningitis** **Encephalitis** **Paralysis** (E.g. Polio) **<u>CHRONIC</u>** **Autism,** **ADHD,** **Alzheimer's,** **M.E., CFS.**
If white blood cells cope with the process very few if any antibodies are produced by the B cells. Remember **ANTIBODIES are FLAGS** to attract other cells.	White cells unable to eliminate what is constantly being flagged by antibodies. So IgE produced to flag toxins as they first contact the body (skin, mouth, upper respiratory etc)	Acute and chronic Inflammatory reactions of the above; **liver, lymphatics, joints, fat, connective tissue, kidneys, heart/valves including glandular fever**.	This may be accompanied by **septicaemic rash. Is NOT an eliminatory rash** but a non-blanching rash indicating internal bleeding seen under the skin (also affects internal organs)

10.4 Understanding infectious illness and susceptibility

We have looked at several issues that help us to understand from a more holistic point of view the nature of what has been called infectious disease and other diseases caused by toxic overload, in summary:

> It is important to separate the 'reaction' from the 'trauma'; successful treatment thereby involves the removal or minimising the trauma whilst also helping the reaction.
> Microbes are often the result of stress/trauma leading to toxic overload and therefore microbes are not the cause.
> It is important to distinguish which symptoms are reactions to trauma and which are consequences, for example the symptoms of vomiting (i.e. elimination of a digestive toxin) and the symptoms of dehydration that could follow if adequate fluid intake is not maintained.
> Once we are aware of the purpose of the symptom reaction, it is vitally important to realise that symptoms can 'succeed' or 'fail', indiscriminately suppressing symptoms will actually predispose one to immune failure.
> Failure of the symptom response leads to symptoms persisting; they do not simply go away, but continue as chronic reactions and potentially deeper chronic disease.
> Chronic disease can therefore have a twofold effect; on the one hand the body is less able to deal with continued trauma and in addition they often allow more of what is traumatic deeper into the system.

The result of 'immune failure' (the failure of the acute reaction to resolve the presenting trauma), is a 'persistent reaction' (i.e. the chronic disease), as such, the factors that determine whether an acute illness resolves or not can be summarised as follows:

1) The amount of trauma that the patient is responding to.
2) The reactive energy /vitality of the patient, i.e. the ability of the patient to respond.
3) The management of their symptoms; in helping or suppressing.

The policy of suppressing immune reactions without addressing underlying causes is responsible for increasing the chronic diseases that we are now witnessing. This can be easily demonstrated by looking at an individual's pattern of disease throughout their life; many patients experience symptoms of allergies, autoimmune disease or more invasive illnesses such as meningitis after vaccines; chronic disease reactions occur after suppressive medication, for example arthritis after suppressing rashes, asthma after suppressing eczema.

This has then been confirmed by looking at the effects on their cellular biochemistry through more detailed research work. In the bigger picture this can also be demonstrated by looking at the epidemiology of disease in populations.

10.5 Suppression and chronic disease – Evidence in the public at large

Jean Francois Bach MD DSc presented a paper in The New England Medical Journal (Vol. 347 No. 12), September 19, 2002, showing that the main factor for the prevalence of allergic and autoimmune disorders is in fact the decrease in infectious diseases. The challenge of reducing such disorders he says is an important one

> "...because of the high morbidity of allergic and autoimmune diseases. In fact, it might extend to other immune disorders, notably non-Hodgkin's lymphomas, the frequency of which is also increasing."

Bach has pieced together the available rates of disease, and his following graphs show clearly the rise in allergic and autoimmune disorders concomitantly with the reduction in infectious diseases.

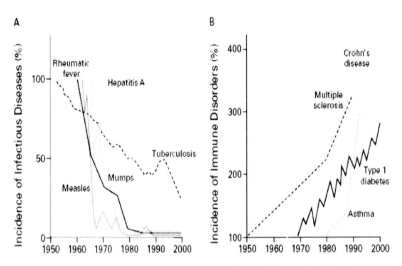

Figure 1. Inverse Relation between the Incidence of Prototypical Infectious Diseases (Panel A) and the Incidence of Immune Disorders (Panel B) from 1950 to 2000.

In Panel A, data concerning infectious diseases are derived from reports of the Centers for Disease Control and Prevention, except for the data on hepatitis A, which are derived from Joussemet et al.[12] In Panel B, data on immune disorders are derived from Swarbrick et al.,[10] Dubois et al.,[13] Tuomilehto et al.,[14] and Pugliatti et al.[15]

Interestingly JF Bach notes these increases in allergic and autoimmune diseases are most significant from 1950 and later, BUT this does not coincide with the decrease in infectious disease which had dramatically declined from 1850 and not from 1950. He does not show how or why this is the case and also does not consider the implications of immune suppression or vaccination.

Decline in infectious disease has been occurring since 1850 not 1950

Whooping Cough

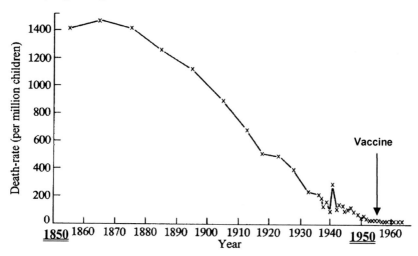

FIGURE 8.12. Whooping cough: death rates of children under 15: England and Wales.

Measles

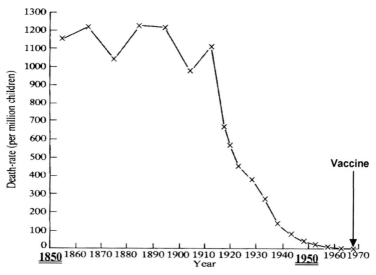

FIGURE 8.14. Measles: death rates of children under 15: England and Wales.

Tuberculosis

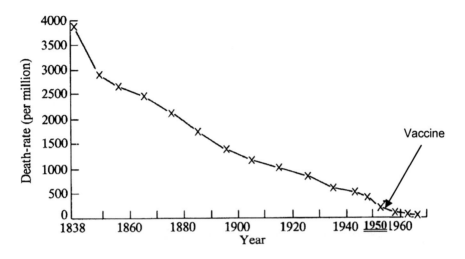

Respiratory TB mean annual death rate England & Wales

Diphtheria

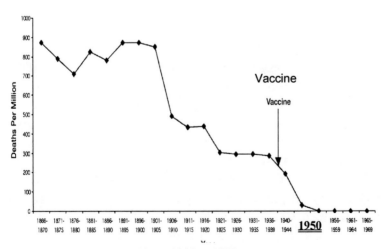

Diphtheria Deaths Per Million Children
(Under 15 years old)

Year: 1865 to 1970

Clearly the rise in allergic and autoimmune diseases cannot be due to the fall in infectious diseases if in fact most of the reduction (over 95% reduction) occurred <u>before</u> 1950 with no concomitant rise in allergic and autoimmune disease. It would therefore appear more significant to look at the impact of procedures more prevalent from the 1950's; this would notably coincide with the increase in use of immune suppressive medication, vaccination and perhaps other environmental poisons, rather than correlated to the decrease in infectious diseases.

10.6 What is the impact of environmental poisons?

By looking at the incidence of asthma we are able to illustrate the significance of individual susceptibility as compared to toxicity. JF Bach in his review article cited above…

> ***"…Even though air pollution can worsen the clinical status of patients with asthma, it does not appear to affect the incidence of asthma. No correlation has been established between pollution indexes and the incidence of asthma.***
>
> *German reunification provided an opportunity to study the effects of air pollution on the development of asthma and atopy (allergy). Several studies found a lower prevalence of asthma, atopic sensitization, and hay fever among residents of cities of the former East Germany, which were more polluted than West German cities. Similarly, the prevalence of asthma in Athens, Greece, is relatively low, despite the high levels of air pollution."*

Therefore the incidence and cause of disease as illustrated by the onset of symptoms in an individual and the prevalence of illness in populations cannot be simply due to the occurrence of pollutants, since **more polluted areas do <u>not</u> have higher incidence of asthmatic disease.** The issue of susceptibility as determined by an individual's previous immune success or failure is actually far more significant and in the developed world this is largely determined by the mode of treatment i.e. the degree of immune suppression, if you want to find allergies and autoimmune disease follow the road of immune suppression.

10.7 Keep doing what you do & you'll keep getting what you get

Without a perspective of:
- Overall immune purpose & function
- The relevance of immune success & failure and
- The relationship between acute & chronic disease.

We are likely to interpret disease simply as some 'thing' that we 'do' or 'do not' have or equally as something that we may 'have had' or 'not have had', from such a limited perspective of disease it may appear self-evident that if we can stop someone producing symptoms of disease, we must therefore have been successful in avoiding disease. The implication is that we are therefore at less risk at suffering the adverse effects of the illness, we have therefore reduced the disease burden and therefore the patient must be potentially healthier. Through such a fragmented perspective of health and illness, conventional scientists are apt to look at the results of Bach and reach conclusions that ultimately twist their theories and practice into mental knots and inconsistencies.

JF Bach therefore comes to the following conclusion...

> There is a certain irony in the fact that we must now search for new ways to reproduce the infectious diseases against which we have been fighting with great success over the past three decades.

Now we are being lead to believe that we have an increased disease burden of allergy and autoimmune disease as a result of our 'successes' in reducing infectious illnesses.

In the restricted view of orthodoxy, the concept of 'success' is simply seen as having fewer apparent symptoms of the original disease;

consequently if it transpires that through such medical intervention (suppression) your health has deteriorated, then you must therefore need more intervention to re-create the original disease.

We know, of course that you can stop someone reacting, but that may in fact make them more susceptible to other more serious disease. With vaccines and other suppressive medication we have created more problems and now we have to search for new ways, (no doubt pharmaceutical ways), to reproduce the original infectious diseases.

> *"...We must now search for new ways to reproduce the infectious diseases against which we have been fighting with great success over the past three decades."*
>
> **JF Bach**

And so we see, as Einstein tells us, 'No problem can ever be solved by the same thinking that created it. We must learn to see the world anew.' However the opposite is being suggested; "...search for new ways to reproduce infectious diseases", is this really the only option?

> *January 2006 study shows reduced allergies without vaccines or the infectious disease rates of the 1950's...*

Further evidence illustrating the error in conventional thinking has been recently obtained from the results of researching 6,600 children reported in the peer reviewed scientific Journal of Allergy & Clinical Immunology in Jan 2006, (Vol.117. No.1). This shows that children of Steiner Schools as compared to other children in the same area were significantly less likely to have allergic conditions such as hayfever, eczema and asthma. Here information on environmental exposure, history of infections, diet, animal contact, lifestyle, and use of medication were studied. Importantly it was found that...

> *Reduced use of antibiotics, antipyretics such as calpol, and reduced MMR vaccine were found to be associated*

with a significant reduction in asthma, eczema and hayfever...

Which is of course entirely predictable if we are able to look at the bigger picture, i.e. stand back and look at the context of our immune reactions and response to pharmaceutical intervention. Vaccines have in fact added to the immune burden and by no means provide the only mechanism for this, there are a vast array of immune suppressive drugs that many people are subjected to; anti-emetics, antipyretics, anti-inflammatories, antihistamines, antibiotics, steroids, bronchodilators, to name but a few.

The immune burden will also be as a result of the toxic burden of which there are a vast array of poisons introduced into our environment, in addition to the nature of nutritional deficiencies as a result of mass farming methods, soil depletion, and the harvesting of foods before ripe to be transported across the world.

Vaccines are, however, exceptionally toxic and by the nature of their administration, being injected into individuals from as young as two months old and in some instances on the first day they are born, vaccines have the potential to be extremely dangerous, especially to individuals who are already immune compromised. To understand the nature of immune compromised individuals, we must be able to understand the consequences of immune success and failure, health is not simply the absence of apparent symptoms. The nature of suppression may also leave periods of reduced symptoms and apparent alleviation but with the 'problem' now manifesting deeper within the individual.

By understanding the nature of physiological responses in disease and the difference between immune success and immune failure, we can chart the course of acute and chronic disease and successfully predict those who are the most susceptible and thereby provide a strategy for cure. It is obvious that some individuals exposed to a potential poison are able to eliminate and keep this out whilst others are not, clearly the immune function of individuals varies enormously, what is poisonous to one is not to another. The results of immune success or failure provide the key to understanding this issue of susceptibility.

We may also inherit certain susceptibilities from our parents, babies are often medicated during the birthing process, given antibiotics for certain discharges, many are fed formula foods, vaccinated, fevers suppressed with antipyretics, eczema treated with immune suppressing steroids, asthma treated likewise with the addition of bronchodilators, allergies treated with anti-histamines, chronic immune conditions with steroidal and non-steroidal anti-inflammatories, each leaving the patient more and more susceptible to environmental toxins, until even their very food becomes an immune burden.

10.8 Medicine – bad for your health

If this were true then the impact of pharmaceutical therapeutics, which is of course separate from accident and emergency care, diagnostics, nutrition and life style care, would on balance be detrimental to the health of a given population: Dr Robert Mendelsohn, author of 'The Medical Heretic' in an article entitled "Staying Healthy In Spite Of Your Doctor" would appear to agree:

> *"I started to collect statistics about doctor's strikes. Whenever doctors stop working, the mortality rate always drops. There are no exceptions to that. In a doctor's strike in Los Angeles, the mortality rate dropped 17%. During an 85 day strike in Israel, the mortality rate dropped 50%, which greatly concerned the morticians, who ran a study of their own and discovered that the last time the mortality rate dropped that low was 20 years previously during the time of the last doctor's strike. So I decided that the recipe for good health was simply retiring all the doctors at full pay, on the condition that they not practice anymore."*

Health would undoubtedly increase if there was a dramatic cut in pharmaceutical drug suppression.

CHAPTER 10 – SUMMARY

> ➢ As a result of immune failure the immune symptoms can persist at a lower level and these reactions continue even though the original stress/trauma is no longer present.
>
> ➢ The consequence of the failure of an inflammatory reaction could be persistent membrane leaking and therefore increased susceptibility to allergens entering the blood.
>
> ➢ If the body is pushed into increased antibody responses that are suppressed and therefore fail, this can also lead to persistent anti-body responses therefore predisposing to allergies and autoimmune disease.
>
> ➢ Internal toxins and complexes of antibodies joined to toxins that are not eliminated affect the internal systems of the body creating more serious internal diseases.
>
> ➢ Vaccines and suppressive medication predispose us to these internalised disease states.
>
> ➢ All of which can be demonstrated in the detailed biochemistry of the person, the individual clinical symptoms of the person and the epidemiology of disease in the wider population.

CHAPTER ELEVEN

11 How do we know whether there has been suppression or cure?

We are aware that there is a place for all kinds of therapeutic intervention, and there will of course be effective and ineffective treatments from all therapeutic systems, there will also be situations where suppressive treatment is appropriate but with regard to the issue of treatment, how do we know what is happening?

If my symptoms are no longer there, has there been suppression or cure? The World Health Organisation is in agreement with the principles of many holistic therapies in acknowledging that health is not simply the absence of *apparent* disease. We know it is possible to remove symptoms through suppression and as a consequence create deterioration in health, it is therefore important to establish criteria we can use to assess the effect of any treatment, (alternative or orthodox), on an individual.

In our assessment of treatment, all of the individual's signs and symptoms, (physically, mentally and emotionally), are paramount, we need to assess the nature of those symptoms as they relate to the whole person and over a significant period of time:

> ➤ Have the presenting symptoms declined?
> ➤ Do they recur at any time in the future and after how long?
> ➤ Are there new symptoms, anywhere else in the body?
> ➤ Do the new symptoms affect more or less important organs?

> ➢ What is the severity of the new symptoms?
> ➢ Is there a resolution of old symptoms from previous illnesses?
> ➢ Does the patient experience more or less limitation now?
> ➢ What is their sense of well-being?
> ➢ How is their mental and emotional state?

Within the field of holistic medicine this subject is studied at great length, we need to know whether there has been a curative response or deterioration. In homeopathy, for example, through the observation of signs and symptoms, criteria have been devised to enable homeopaths to discern if the response to treatment has been curative and whether previous issues have been suppressed or resolved.

The pattern of symptom response that indicates a curative reaction has been well established, it was originally systematised by the homeopath Constantine Hering and revised by others since, but is still referred to as Hering's Law of Cure and is used by many kinds of therapists. This basically states that in a curative reaction symptoms move from top to bottom, from inside to out, from more important organs to less important organs, in reverse order of appearance, and later added from tissues of the later evolved embryonic germ layers to earlier germ layers. A similar formulation has also been established by the naturopaths and their training often includes the principles of Constantine Hering. Naturopaths work very closely with osteopaths, for a long time their training involved both disciplines. Practitioners of Traditional Chinese Medicine also make observations that correlate diverse aspects of the body and mind in their assessment of cure.

These criteria stem from the research of observable reactions in many individuals comparing those experiencing curative reactions to those where there is deterioration. This then leads us to a study of the nature and pattern of illness, not only within the lifetime of an individual, but also over successive generations.

11.1 Interpreting Patterns of Illness as a method of determining suppression or cure - The Significance of Acute & Chronic Disease

As previously described, we have distinguished four approximate outcomes to an acute disease as follows:

1. The individual resolves the illness and as a result, the health is improved and they are stronger than they were before. They are then less susceptible to those problems after the illness and more able to deal with them.
2. The individual resolves the illness but there has been no learning as such, they are not stronger than they were before, they effectively carry on, as they were before the illness, just as susceptible to succumbing to the illness as they were before.
3. The illness is not resolved and as a result, the health of the individual is worse than before and they descend into a lower level of chronic illness, and therefore more susceptible to the same problem than they were before.
4. The illness is not resolved and the patient is unable to react sufficiently to overcome the problem and dies.

And similarly we can illustrate diagrammatically the nature of these patterns, enabling us to see the effect of disease and treatment, with regard to the overall health of the patient.

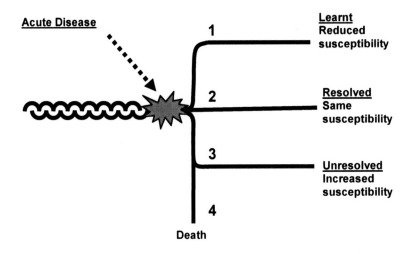

Acute Disease

1

Learnt
Reduced
susceptibility

2

Resolved
Same
susceptibility

3

Unresolved
Increased
susceptibility

4

Death

11.2 The value of acute disease in the chronically ill

Let us further imagine a situation where somebody already has a chronic illness and exists on level 3 above. We could use our simple example of a child that suffers an acute grief from the separation trauma of their first day at nursery, a grief that is not resolved because of an initial suppression, perhaps told off for crying or told off for over-reacting and so develops a chronic sadness.

In the chronic illness we observe symptoms (sadness) that are **similar** to the acute symptoms (crying) but are **less intense** and last for **longer**. On the face of it, the acute grief has been stopped, however the child is now **more susceptible** to suffering and has become sensitised to those kinds of traumas (separation), the disease so to speak has not been resolved but suppressed. Later we may see that the child becomes upset when the parents leave the room in their home even if close by in another room, the child is more sensitive to separation as a result of the unresolved grief, its susceptibility has increased.

How are they to resolve this sadness? Well it is likely that any similar reaction to another trauma could result in another acute reaction that actually helps to resolve the underlying sadness and brings them back up to a higher level of health than before. So the mother, leaving the child in a room on their own, an issue that would previously have been ok is now problematic, this leads to a grief reaction and the child will in fact be reacting to the presenting issue plus the underlying unresolved issue. On the face of it the child appears to be over-reacting, which is somehow indicative of our propensity to judge critically the workings of the human being if they do not appear to be operating within our designated 'norm'. The reaction is however appropriate to the presenting issue plus the underlying unresolved issue, the camel's back appears to break from the last straw, but does of course break from the accumulated weight of all the previous straws. If the recent grief reaction is allowed expression this could be enough to resolve the present and underlying issue, the child feels better and is now back to their previous level of health.

11.3 The management of acute symptoms has pivotal implications to overall health.

The level of trauma needed to create this second reaction would be less than the original trauma, as the child is already sensitised. However, in order to resolve this second acute and subsequently the underlying chronic condition such that the child's level of health is increased, one would have to address the initial factors that lead to the child dropping into the chronic illness in the first place. In that particular instance the problem was the suppression, if this is not addressed i.e. if the child is not allowed to express their grief in the subsequent trauma then there may be further consequences; the system could be maintained at that same chronic level, similar state of sadness and therefore susceptible to recurrent reactions or it could be further compromised and the child could slip further into a deeper chronic illness.

At a deeper level of illness, similar traumas to that of the initial grief may not now be able to stimulate sufficient reaction to resolve the initial problem and in fact the child would now be desensitised to the initial kinds of traumatic events. This lower level of chronic illness will invariably take on a different character to the previous one and could for example create chronic irritability, anger or timidity depending on the individual nature of the child.

Thereby we can imagine how individuals can exist at various levels of health according to their history of either resolution of illness or deterioration. It is interesting to consider the Hermetic dictum "as above, so below" when viewing health in terms of energetic levels. Our health therefore appears to jump in levels, up or down at points of crisis known as our acute disease and interesting that our physical structure as delineated by atoms, contain particles that will equally jump from one level to another and do not exist in all possible states in a linear progression. These sub-atomic 'particles' will absorb energy and vibrate with higher energy but do not jump to higher levels until they have received a sufficient quantum of energy.

Likewise it appears that we can increase our general vitality but need to experience an acute reaction in order to transform health and therefore reduce susceptibility to illness, consequently the management of acute disease has pivotal implications to overall health.

From this simplified scheme it is possible to see the purpose of the acute illness not only in reacting to the presenting problem but also in resolving the underlying chronic pattern of illness. With many of us carrying unresolved physical and emotional issues, our reactions to life events are very rarely reactions to just that presenting event.

From the following diagram and what we have discussed earlier we can also see that the resolution of a particular trauma actually makes us LESS susceptible to those events afterwards – a degree of immunity, so to speak, and our level of health increases, as we would experience through any learning process.

11.3.1 Resolution of acute illness

We can therefore see the positive value in overcoming a particular trauma, if we already have a chronic illness i.e. an existing sensitivity, (here sensitivity refers to the ease at which you are <u>adversely</u> affected by a trauma/substance <u>not</u> a measure of awareness). A successful reaction in the acute illness would help to overcome the presenting issue <u>and</u> the underlying chronic, which will thereby lead to an increased level of health.

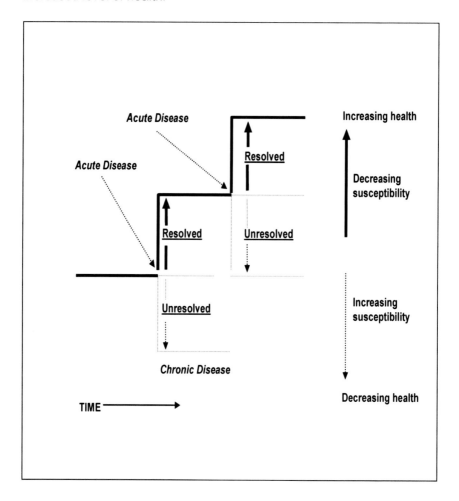

11.3.2 Unresolved acute illness

Conversely unresolved illnesses may lead to chronic conditions and if further acute reactions are not resolved this may lead to deeper chronic disease.

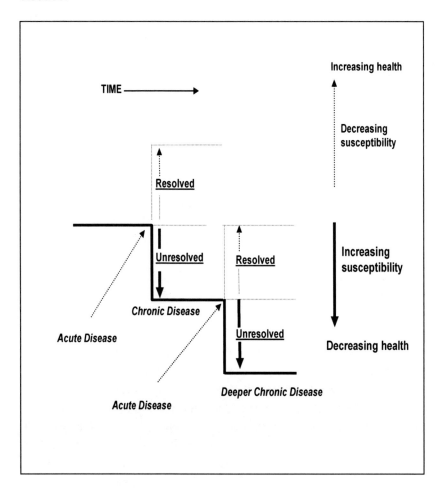

Dr Thomas Quak in his article 'Vaccinations and their side-effects' notes the phenomenon of acute illness resolving chronic and the often reported incidence of childhood illnesses leading to developmental leaps:

> In Annals of Tropical Paediatrics, (Chakravarti, V.S. and Lingam, S., "Measles induced remission of psoriasis, 1986, 6; pages 293-294) the following case is reported:
>
> 1984 a 5 year-old girl presented with a bad case of psoriasis. She showed large affected areas on her body and extremities, also involving to a significant degree her scalp. During the following year she was treated by Paediatricians and Dermatologists with coal tar preparations, local steroids, UV light, and dithranol wraps. Despite these therapies and two hospitalizations, the **psoriasis was refractory and remained essentially unchanged** until she came down with measles. As the **measles rash began to spread over her skin, the psoriasis disappeared**. Since then she has been free of psoriasis.

It is therefore possible to map the progress of acute and chronic illness, moving up and down the levels of health according to resolution or suppression. The further up you exist the greater the level of health and the less susceptible you are to illness, the wider tolerance you have to your environment and therefore the more adaptable you are. In situations of high stress, e.g. injury, poisoning etc, you could still succumb to a condition that you are unable to overcome and die, but you would be able to withstand much more trauma than on the lower levels, and therefore suppression of your reaction would not help but hinder your attempt at resolution.

Health on the lower levels is more restricted, being more sensitised with less reactive energy, generally poorer immune function and greater levels of toxicity that are more invasive into the body. The lower your level of health, the more these problems are exacerbated, consequently it takes less stress to upset these individuals and they are therefore closer to serious disease and are already suffering chronic conditions.

Given the ability to map illnesses as such, we can see how different individuals on the various levels are in fact susceptible to different kinds of illnesses. With regard to infectious disease this is particularly enlightening as we can see that contrary to popular belief, contraction of a so-called infectious illness is not simply a matter of an indiscriminate hit by a microbe or group of them. This is why most individuals in contact with others that have an infectious disease do not succumb to that illness and that many individuals with the same microbial illness can have vastly differing symptom pictures. We are only susceptible to certain illnesses according to our particular state e.g. glandular, lung, skin etc and in each area of susceptibility symptoms may be very mild affecting external systems or more severe affecting more internal systems.

The acute reaction therefore gives us the opportunity to resolve chronic issues, if we are able to support the individual and their dis-ease reactions.

11.4 However, what of the value of chronic disease?

"Considering the alternative it's not too bad at all"

Maurice Chevalier in his response to old age

The answer to any question of benefit lies in the consideration of available alternatives in any given situation. If during an acute illness our reactions are not sufficiently strong enough to resolve the trauma, then the body cannot sustain that level of reaction indefinitely; the nature of the acute reaction is intense and therefore can only be short-lived. As a consequence, the failure to react sufficiently will lead to a continued reduced reaction that is however more sustainable over a longer period of time, this is our chronic condition, a persistent reaction over a longer duration, the energy of which would not be sufficient however to resolve the trauma. If this chronic reaction did not to happen, the reaction of the body during an acute would continue at a high intensity and if unsuccessful there would be no halfway house, the individual would die.

Therefore the chronic disease is in fact the next best thing, given an unsuccessful response to a trauma; it demonstrates the forgiving and compromising nature of the human body, always attempting to sustain life. If chronic disease were not an option there would be far fewer of us on the planet, but yes…we'd be healthier! You would either succeed or die; however this does not appear to be a feature of life.

For example if an acute rash did not resolve the internal blood toxicity, rather than continue in an acute generalised inflammatory state you may develop a chronic rash, less intense reaction that continues for longer. An acute cough could become a chronic asthma, vomiting and diarrhoea become persistent nausea, acute emotional reactions become chronic sadness, but also affecting specific organs.

It is interesting to note how commentaries on modern medicine suggest that the success of medical intervention has enabled us to sustain very sick individuals that in nature would have died; a survival of the fittest philosophy that we are possibly going against, we are victims of our own medical success. However this does emanate from a misguided and arrogant interpretation of our abilities in medicine. Although undeniably we are able to perform remarkable technological feats in terms of keeping individuals alive, medical technology has <u>not</u> been applied to creating health, but is in fact obsessively suppressing intelligent healing responses whilst on the other hand technologically advanced in holding together the pieces of those damaged human beings.

Cancers, autoimmune disease, allergies, autism, cardio-vascular disease are in fact all increasing with the advent of our modern technological advances.

➢ Dr. Samuel S. Epstein: Emeritus Professor, Environmental and Occupational Medicine University of Illinois School of Public Health and Chairman, Cancer Prevention Coalition. www.preventcancer.com

> *A report from the World Health Organization's International Agency for Research on Cancer (IARC), published in the current issue of the International Journal of Cancer, January 2002;97:72-81 confirms that the crude prevalence of overall and organ-specific **cancers in men and women is higher in developed than in developing nations**.*

One could also assume that the rise in chronic disease in developed countries could be a result of increased life expectancy leading to more old people and consequently more old age disease. This does not explain the increase in degenerative childhood disease but more importantly does not explain why the developed nations spending more on dealing with cancer, for example, have the most cancer:

> *Among developed nations, the highest prevalence is in the U.S., followed by Western Europe, Australia and New Zealand.*

> *It should be stressed that incidence is the major determinant of crude cancer prevalence, so that regional and national variations reflect variations in risk, and thus avoidable causes of cancer. **That the U.S. invidiously leads the world in this respect is troubling, and is in inverse relationship to the massive public and private funding of the U.S. cancer establishment**, the National Cancer Institute, and American Cancer Society, compared to relatively low funding in other developed nations and regions.*

➢ British Medical Journal July 8, 2000: 321: 88-92. The number of adults suffering from asthma has more than doubled in the last 2 decades, with steroid prescriptions increasing 6-fold.

The main reason for the asthma increase is allergies. Among people who never smoked the rate of hay fever (a type of allergy) went up from 6% to 20% and the rate of asthma increased from 3% to 8%. Among smokers, hay fever rose from 5% to 16% and asthma went up from 2% to 5%. The number of prescriptions for inhaled steroid medications for asthma has increased more than 6 times in the last decade.

➤ Ramyani Gupta et al, reports in the BMJ 2003: 327:1142-1143 (15 November),

Epidemiological studies indicate that the prevalence of allergic disorders such as allergic rhinitis, asthma, and eczema have increased during recent decades in many Western countries.

➤ On the subject of life threatening allergic responses a European Allergy White Paper: 'Allergic diseases as a public health problem' by UCB Institute of Allergy, 2004, suggests these too are on the increase.

Highly significant increases in admissions for systemic allergic diseases (anaphylaxis, angio-oedema, food allergy, and urticaria) occurred in England between 1990-1 and 2000-1. This almost certainly reflects an increase in incidence.

➤ Regarding autoimmune diseases U.S. National Institutes of Health, Autoimmune Diseases Coordinating Committee report in March 2005 in their paper 'Progress in Autoimmune Diseases Research'

... Collectively they affect 14.7 to 23.5 million people in this country, and – for reasons unknown – their prevalence is rising.

Many of these illnesses affect children and young adults and are therefore not as a result of chronic diseases in an older population. In fact much of our increase in life-expectancy has been due to the reduced incidence of childhood deaths over the last century as opposed to adults living longer, significantly experts are predicting that our actual longevity may have started to decline.

➤ S. Jay Olshansky et al in the New England Journal of Medicine, March 17, 2005 (Vol. 352: 1138-1145, No. 11).

> *From our analysis of the effect of obesity on longevity, we conclude that the steady rise in life expectancy during the past two centuries may soon come to an end.*

CHAPTER 11 - SUMMARY

> ➢ It is important to be able to assess whether the outcome of your disease process (treated or not) has led to deterioration or resolution (suppressed or not).
> ➢ There are observable signs that indicate suppression or cure.
> ➢ If disease is resolved we have learnt and are less susceptible, if resolved and not learnt susceptibility is the same, if unresolved we are more susceptible.
> ➢ In chronic disease, acute reactions help to resolve presenting stress/trauma as well as underlying issues that have not yet been resolved.
> ➢ Management of acute disease is therefore pivotal to overall heath.
> ➢ Chronic diseases are persisting acute reactions but at a much lower intensity. They occur if the acute reactions were not strong enough to deal with a stress/trauma, they will continue even if the trauma is no longer there.
> ➢ Chronic disease reactions can also occur if we are subjecting ourselves to a persistent and mild stress/trauma, remove the stress/trauma and the chronic reaction stops.

CHAPTER TWELVE

12 Inherited patterns of disease

Why do some children seem to start off in life with so many health issues?

We are now able to take the story further still, if any chronic disease persists long enough in an individual the whole human-being (mentally, emotionally and physically) will be affected, the individual learns to live within the confines of their condition, until eventually they are <u>unlikely</u> to be able, or even want to react and elevate themselves out of that chronic condition and therefore <u>unable</u> to resolve these limitations to an increased level of health. They may be able to live fairly full lives within those boundaries, however the sensitivities will remain and the individual learns adaptive behaviour to avoid the situations that they feel they are unable to cope with. In homeopathic terms this is effectively known as the <u>miasm</u> – the acquired chronic disease pattern that reflects physiological, mental and emotional limitations of the individual that usually will only be seen under stress.

Now the interesting question for us is what happens if this individual was to have a child? From the observation of these chronic disease patterns from over 200 years of homeopathic treatment, it has become quite clear that these patterns are in fact passed on to the next generation. This is termed the <u>inherited miasm</u> and is a very important concept in homeopathy and holistic practices; the patterns of illness in the parents allow the practitioner insight into the nature of the child's underlying susceptibilities and the likely course of events that will follow successful treatment or suppression.

If we recall from our preceding discussion, a curative response enables the patient to resolve conditions that have been previously suppressed and therefore the patient experiences a return of old symptoms, these symptoms are not necessarily as acute as they were and can often be very fleeting representations of old unresolved conditions.

> *For example in an individual with chronic eczema and food intolerances after the use of hydrocortisone on the skin rash this suppresses the skin elimination of blood toxins and could cause the individual to localise the blood toxins in the joints with concomitant arthritic pains and inflammation. With a more holistic therapeutic intervention successfully treating the joint problems we would expect the rash to return, which would be a sign that the patient is following the direction of cure. Continued treatment of the returned rash would see the rash disappear from the upper parts of the body to the lower parts leaving the patient cured and less sensitised to their food and environmental pollutants.*

By distinguishing and classifying these patterns of chronic disease (inherited and acquired miasms) practitioners are able to predict: how deep a problem is, what areas need to be addressed first, what symptoms to expect during a curative response and what problems lie immediately ahead if illnesses are not resolved (i.e. suppressed).

Therefore an individual with inherited patterns of illness will need to resolve issues that relate to the unresolved issues of their parents, consequently a very important point to appreciate is that we don't all start off with a clean slate, we are not all born equal. The child's physical, mental and emotional state will be compromised by the inherited patterns of unresolved conditions of the parents; this is perfectly illustrated in the observation of dis-ease patterns after curative treatment, the patient experiences patterns of illnesses of previous generations.

By way of example, if asthmatic parents were to have a child, the child could inherit what homeopaths call a tubercular pattern (involving the lymphatics and lungs) which wouldn't necessarily directly translate to asthma but could for example give rise to the tendency to have enlarged tonsils, a sensitivity to milk creating respiratory congestion, colds that quickly lead to coughs, in addition to specific fears and psychological traits. Acute coughs and inflamed tonsils if treated holistically could allow the child to resolve those conditions and may then enable the child to have acute eliminative rashes instead of toxins building up more internally in the lymphatic tissue, rashes that would have been less likely than before. However, suppress the inherited lymphatic reactions and the child could develop deeper illnesses perhaps in the lungs or even glandular fever, chronic fatigue and so on.

The sins of the father are visited on the son... so to speak. Although this rather patriarchal saying has forgotten that we also have mothers! Therefore it is further complicated by the fact that an individual will have two parents and consequently different possibilities of inherited miasms. From the observation of these inherited patterns it is apparent that a child may take on more of the miasm of one parent or the other or from both, so that children within the same family can actually inherit different characteristics in terms of illness patterns. It appears, however, that they cannot start off at the higher levels indicative of resolved health if neither parent has resolved those issues.

Similarly if the next generation are unable to resolve these inherited issues and in fact create further unresolved issues then these deeper miasms are passed on to the next generation and so on. It is important to distinguish that the inherited miasm relates to the pattern of illness as distinguished by chronic disease patterns including physical, mental and emotional symptoms and not just the specific illness from an orthodox medical diagnosis.

For example eczema although one type of chronic illness can be different according to the different miasms, it can occur only in certain circumstances, or with certain foods, or in the folds of elbows and knees, or in other patterns cover much larger areas of the body. Similarly one inherited miasm, for example one that we will call the tubercular miasm, may be associated with different illnesses, tonsillitis, asthma, eczema, hayfever, behavioural tantrums, etc. all apparently different conditions but given other characteristics may all be from the same miasm.

Interestingly these observations are being confirmed by other holistic therapists in their treatment and assessment of patients with chronic disease: Dr Dietrich Klinghardt uses family constellation work to deal with these inherited patterns from previous generations:

> *"Unresolved trauma doesn't simply go away with their death but it plays out in a variety of different ways in later generations and often becomes the cause of illness generations later. Most people overlook this and can never help their patients. One of my major contributions is, I use this work in all of my autistic patients that come to me. The vulnerability that these children have is not only explained on vaccines, mercury and electromagnetic effects, things that we know for sure contribute to autism, but it also has a base in the family history, when we can resolve issues in the family history there is often magical improvements in these children.*

There are, of course, more detailed descriptions of the symptoms, names and classification of miasms, which would be the scope of a more in depth study and there are many standard homeopathic text books on the subject. However, the principle of acquired and inherited chronic disease and therefore miasmatic theory in its basic form is a simple but important concept to grasp.

Therefore to summarise, if acute illnesses are not resolved then persistent reactions will remain, this is the chronic disease. This eventually affects the susceptibility of the whole person and is called the acquired miasm, if not resolved this pattern of acquired miasm will be then passed on to their children which is called the inherited miasm.

12.1 Genetics

Cellular biologists and biochemists have discovered that the genes of each of your cells, (made up of DNA), are the physical components that code for how the various structures of the cells are made and therefore how each cell looks and functions. These genetic codes are copied during cell division and these genes retain the memory of the characteristics of the previous generation.

It is the genes given to you from your parents that determine your characteristics and therefore the reason for the similarities that a child has to their parents. There are of course differences in children from the same parents partly due to the random mixing of genes that you receive from both parents.

It had been assumed for many years that these genetic codes were fixed and unchangeable. Classical Darwinian evolution suggested that improvements to the genetic code, resulting in some enhancement of the function and survivability of the species was a random chance event that could not be specifically predetermined by any individual or their environment.

Similarly, if there was a specific problem with your genetic code, there was nothing you could do to fix it, nothing you could do to avoid the consequences of that defective code and nothing you could do that could reduce the likelihood of creating any future genetic defect. Although there are known chemicals and types of radiation that can increase the likelihood of genetic changes, these were random changes that more often than not lead to the damage of the genetic code.

It was known that some illnesses appeared to be caused by a defect in the genetic code and it was then assumed that these defects and hopefully many more mal-functions could be addressed by simply manipulating the genes. Disease due to genetic defects were therefore thought to be the remit of genetic engineering only, due to the belief that it was impossible to change your genes through any natural, environmental or lifestyle intervention.

It was therefore deduced that any genetic problem could only have been initiated by chance and subsequently passed on to unfortunate individuals of successive generations. Generally these genetic defects would have been caused by very potent toxins called mutagens, damaging radiation or a mishap in the replication process.

Therefore, according to classical genetics, it is not possible to initiate a coordinated change in your genes by the events that happen in one's own life. Consequently it would appear that the observations of holistic therapists, whereby unresolved illnesses in one's lifetime could affect the inherited characteristics of your children, are not in keeping with the science of genetics. However, genetic understanding has now developed considerably and is now, in fact, more in keeping with the observations of holistic therapists.

The genes contain much of the inherited information and modern scientists now know that the initial dogma whereby the environment cannot influence the genes is wrong. Although once the pattern (miasm) has been ingrained, hard-wired so to speak, it is difficult to shift, but depending on the degree of hard wiring, it is possible to change.

12.2 What controls the controllers?

It is important to recognise that every single cell inside the body (apart from cells that have lost their nucleus e.g. mature red blood cells and the reproductive cells, sperm and eggs), although widely different in function, appearance and physiology, carries exactly the same genetic information, cells of the stomach wall, liver, eye, nerves, bones etc. all contain exactly the same genes. Biochemists and geneticists are aware that if the mere presence of genes were solely responsible for the characteristics of the cells then all of our cells would be the same and quite clearly they are not.

Therefore, even if genes could not change, more important than the presence of genes would be the question of what determines the expression of genes in different cells. There is an incredible variety of expression due to the switching on, or off, of specific genes and the fact that a single gene can be used in a variety of ways. Therefore the most significant differences may not be what genes you have or don't have but which genes are switched on or off and in what manner are these genes being used in any given situation i.e. what is controlling these genes. Hence the new discipline of **epigenetics**, the study of the controlling influences of other molecules and external factors on gene expression.

Furthermore the material that is transferred between each parent to create the unborn child, the fusion of sperm cell and ova to form the fertilised egg, consists of more than just genes. Even from that most basic point of view, clearly not all of the physical inheritance is contained in the genes. Bruce Lipton in his book 'The Biology of Belief' quotes from biologist Marion Lamb and philosopher Eva Jablonka:

> *"In recent years, molecular biology has shown that the genome is far more fluid and responsive to the environment than previously supposed. It has also shown that information can be transmitted to descendants in ways other than through the base sequence of DNA" (i.e. other than through the genes)*

'Epigenetic inheritance and Evolution – The Lamarckian Dimension'
(1995) Marion Lamb & Eva Jablonka.

Of what significance are these ideas in modern genetics? Bruce Lipton is a modern scientist passionate about the significance of recent discoveries made in cellular biology.

> *"My career as a biomedical research scientist began in 1967 when I started cloning stem cells, years before conventional*

science was aware of their importance in human health. While a tenured member of the University of Wisconsin's Medical School faculty, I was involved with teaching each new crop of medical students the basic science of how cells work."

Bruce Lipton

Like many geneticists Bruce Lipton taught the central dogma, basically once you had inherited your genes, then that was that, the inherited program (the genetic program) would, from then on, determine how you functioned and ultimately how you behaved in your life. These genes could not be changed unless affected in some chance biochemical accident or similarly by the chance effect of some mutagenic poison. You are victims of your genes and therefore sickness could ultimately be linked to a defective gene, if we could fix the gene we could cure the sickness. However, Bruce Lipton, like other scientists, was soon to discover quite the opposite.

"While I was teaching the Dogma in class, my cloned human cells began to reveal a completely different story. Rather than genes, the experiments revealed that it was the environment that was 'controlling' the cells. By changing the environmental conditions within the culture dish, the same cells could be transformed to reveal radically different expressions.

And by my questioning the Dogma of gene-control, I was labelled a heretic and actually shunned by my colleagues...Religious belief aside, there is a fundamental question that must be asked, "Do genes really control biology?" The answer to that question is unambiguously, NO. This fact was scientifically established by the late 1980's, when a new awareness arose in molecular biology. That awareness provided for one of today's most active areas of scientific research, the field of epigenetics. Epigenetics is a study of the molecular mechanisms by which environment controls gene activity."

*In 1988, a Harvard geneticist and biochemist named John Kearns published in Scientific American, perhaps the most important paper in the history of biology. He countered the idea of random cellular mutation as set forth by Darwin with the idea of specific mutation brought on by the conditions of the environment. The implications are enormous, establishing the primacy of the environment over genetic determinacy…This body of work in fact proves that cells are regulated by responses to the environment. **Genes are not causative, but only correlated,** just blueprints that are altered as needed by environmental demands.*

Because we do in fact respond to our environment on the fundamental level of genes, research indicates that it is therefore not just the environment but our perception of the environment that we are responding to, this lead Bruce Lipton on the quest to establish therefore how do our beliefs and perceptions affect who we are, how do they affect our genes and therefore our physical bodies and what can we do to enhance physical, mental and emotional health.

*"Frontier research in cell biology has finally acknowledged the mechanisms by which perception controls behaviour, selects genes and can even lead to a rewriting of the genome. Rather than being the victims of our genes, we have been the victims of our perceptions! ... We are beginning to realize that **transforming our lives is a lot easier than rewriting our genetic code or addicting ourselves to drugs."***

Bruce Lipton

"Life is a movie you see through your own unique eyes .It makes little difference what's happening out there. It's how you take it that counts."

Denis Waitley

It appears that there are many factors that can affect genes, environmental and behavioural factors, even our own perceptions, and we know that these factors can also change the predisposition to illness and therefore the miasmatic patterns of illness. People can and do evolve to be sicker as well as evolve to be healthier, it is not only the fit that survive, but the slightly less fit, right down to the completely incapacitated, and that's not only because we are keeping sick people alive, but as a direct result of making them sick. The survival of the fittest doctrine of Darwinian Evolution; creating ever healthier individuals and eliminating the weaker ones, only holds true if slight encumbrances are always eliminated and do not breed, which of course is not the case, even in the natural world.

There are many new and interesting discoveries that have led to a reconsideration of classical Darwinian evolution; inherent in classical evolution is the idea that increased adaptation occurred by chance and was naturally selected for, (chance mutation and natural selection). That is, organisms had to wait around for aeons until, by chance, some mutagenic chemical or photon of radiation bumped into a piece of DNA in the genetic code and inadvertently changed it in such a manner that the new DNA coded for a new cellular property that enabled you to survive better than all of your pals. So much so that all of your peers could not compete with you and consequently died off, 'natural selection'.

The natural world was a harsh competitive environment that naturally selected for the fittest and quickly eliminated the weak; this is of course a hypothesis that reflects a belief system as much as one that reflects the facts. It encompasses the idea of scarce resources that need to be competed for, with the prize of survival to the victor and death to loser, having no guiding principle other than pure chance.

There are of course many problems with this theory but we shall look at a couple of aspects and realise how new facts may change ones outlook. Firstly we now know that this process will be infinitely speeded up if in fact individuals can directly adapt to their environment, they do not have to wait for 'chance mutations' to change things, but can directly adapt optimally to their environmental conditions. In addition, if cellular adaptation, information and gene transfer can be transferred across to other cells and other individuals, therefore not just via inheritance down the line to offspring, then evolution does not have to wait for the products of reproduction. Consequently evolution can occur more quickly and we appear to be directed by our environment including all life in our environment, competition for resources (although may be present) is not in fact the major force directing evolution and cooperation appears to be much more important given the interdependency of environment, food, waste-products and organic life forms.

> *"When Charles Darwin wrote his thesis about evolution and the survival of the fittest, another man Peter Kropotkin of Russia was writing quite a diametrically opposite thesis that evolution happens through cooperation... The very idea that one evolves through conflict is violent; it is a very lopsided idea... The Darwinian vision is a very inhuman meditation about life... Violence may be a part but it is not the whole; deep down is cooperation. And the higher you grow the less and less violence the more and more cooperation there is. That is the ladder of growth."*
>
> **Osho**

Significantly therefore, enhanced adaptability is only possible if we are allowed to adapt, i.e. allowed to respond, if in fact we are suppressing responses then it is ill-health and restricted adaptability that we are inheriting.

As such, the concept of miasm, (acquired and inherited chronic disease) is deduced from observable phenomena, i.e. from the observation of patterns of disease as a consequence of resolved or unresolved diseases. From the detailed observation of these patterns of illness we are then able to predict the consequences of successful or suppressive treatment. We are therefore not limiting ourselves to the relatively small proportion of illnesses that can be correlated to the classical genetic blueprints, as this discovery itself still leaves us short of explaining why the patient has the genetic blueprint for the disease and what to do about it.

We now know that elements other than 'chance' affect genes and so in discovering genetic blueprints to an individual's illness we now have to consider what factors predisposed that patient to the genetic disease, what causes those genetic 'adaptations', pure chance, environmental stress, symptom suppression etc. We are therefore challenged to find ways to treat the presenting illness and of equal importance, investigate predisposing factors that create those genetic tendencies so that we are able to reduce the likelihood of those conditions for the benefit of future generations.

Therapists have known that many disease patterns are inherited conditions long before geneticists are able to find the specific gene or other biochemical markers of inheritance, the important thing is to know what conditions produce the disease pattern in the first place, what triggers the expression of a dormant disease pattern and more importantly how do we resolve the condition in individuals.

The biochemical detail may eventually provide some clues but so far much of the relevant story has already been exposed by looking at the bigger picture. Geneticists have been able to identify disease blueprints in the form of genes in individuals, but the inherited condition can already be known by looking at the patterns of disease in the individual and their previous generations, geneticists in spite of deciphering the complete human genome have yet to apply that knowledge to anything useful in the arena of health and illness. Dr. Peter P. Gariaev, Ph.D. of the Russian Academy of Natural Sciences:

> *"Paradoxically, the more success we have in such genetics and molecular biology technologies, the farther we seem to be from understanding the actual foundational principles, the inner workings, of the genetic codes. With our present understanding, we cannot cure cancer, we cannot resist AIDS, we have not defeated tuberculosis, nor can we at present*

prolong significantly the lives of people. Initial promises of a bright future, based on creations of trans-genetic research, have actually turned out to be only dangerous trans-genetic foodstuffs, hazardous to the biosphere on which our very lives depend. The cloning of animals has produced only ugly and useless creatures, or animals that grow old and die abnormally rapidly, as in the well-known case of the cloned sheep, Dolly. And it is quite natural that these results cause alarm within the scientific community".

Genetic research has yet to be able to treat any condition inherited or otherwise, whereas other therapies already can.

CHAPTER 12 - SUMMARY

> Patterns of chronic disease that remain in an individual for sustained periods of time become more hard-wired so to speak and the individual learns adaptive behaviour to avoid the situations that they feel they are unable to cope with.

> This chronic disease pattern is known as the <u>miasm</u> – the acquired pattern that reflects physiological, mental and emotional limitations of the individual that will usually only be seen under stress.

> These patterns of disease can be passed on from one generation to the next and therefore illnesses in the affected children will reflect their own stresses plus the underlying issues that were not dealt with by their parents.

> The factors predisposing us to inherited disease can be researched and therefore reduced and/or avoided. Labelling a disease as genetic does not absolve us of responsibility for reducing the incidence of that disease.

> Likewise inherited patterns of disease can also be addressed in a similar manner to acquired chronic diseases, albeit with more difficulty.

CHAPTER THIRTEEN

13 The psychological consequences of suppression

Returning to the principle of the 'suppression' of symptoms in the treatment of disease, it may still be possible to demonstrate some value in suppressive medication. For example this strategy could slow down a process and could, if the practitioner is aware of the underlying issues, create time by delaying resolution, and at some point later allow a more curative treatment and lifestyle adjustment. The major difficulty with pharmaceutical suppression however lays in its lack of perspective i.e. its lack of understanding of what suppression is and this approach being its **only** approach.

During pharmaceutical treatment, suppression is not balanced with a 'recognition' of the need to deal with the underlying causation of the illness, nor will it be recognised that the process could be a necessary learning experience for the body and therefore an opportunity to increase its ability to adapt.

We have discussed the consequences of investing in suppressive treatments as a result of viewing the 'disease symptom' as the 'problem' (instead of the reaction to the problem), predisposing individuals to deeper ailments and more chronic disease; however, on closer investigation, we can see there are perhaps even more profound issues at stake.

What are the psychological differences that occur when we compare a more holistic approach to an orthodox drug approach and how do they ultimately lead to differences in the development of our belief systems and future strategies for living? Our deeds are determined by our perceptions; whether we use an antique table for interior design, a work bench, an opportunity to trade & make money or for fire-wood, is firstly a consequence of perception.

HOLISTIC (non-suppressive)	ORTHODOX (suppressive)
Symptoms are seen as intelligent, beneficial and an essential part of the curative response.	Symptoms seen as a malfunction.
Intervention designed to help the individual to do what they are already doing, i.e. to aid the symptom response; this places more faith in the ability of the patient.	Taught that malfunction will inevitably get worse, therefore the need to suppress is ultimately based on fear and worst case scenarios.
The response is enhanced and therefore our ability to respond is enhanced, therefore less likely to need further intervention.	Response is suppressed and our ability to respond deteriorates, more likely to need further intervention.
Symptom response requires us to understand what we are responding to, therefore addresses the causes.	Not usually correlated to what we are responding to and the cause is not addressed.
Correlations are made with how we are individually affected by the environment around us and therefore we are able to understand our own unique susceptibilities.	Causation not often linked to environment but treatment focuses on the symptom reaction in isolation, no inclination to understand how we are affected by our environment.
Psychologically empowered to make changes to help ourselves and to trust our reactions as they are beneficial aspects of cure.	Psychologically disempowered, taught that your body goes wrong, the only effective intervention is from external drug and expert Dr.
Leads to increased self-knowledge, enhanced ability and trust in oneself.	Leads to fear, dependence on drugs and doctors, with reduced trust in oneself.

The basis of the orthodox model has far reaching implications regarding the outcome of our perceptions regarding health and illness. Signs and symptoms of disease become reasons to be fearful, there appears to be no emphasis on positive outcomes and no prospect of learning, the expert is someone other than you and your salvation lies in the effectiveness of a suppressive drug, a drug to which you could become ultimately dependent.

Slowly but surely responsibility for your health is taken away from you and for many it is willingly surrendered, illness is seen as a mal-function or a condition that is caused by dangerous microbes and it has nothing to do with 'you'. The power to heal, to adapt and survive, slowly erodes, whilst financial resources accumulate from the general public into the hands of very few.

13.1 Placebo

> *"The greatest mistake in the treatment of diseases is that there are physicians for the body and physicians for the soul, although the two cannot be separated."*
>
> **Plato**

From the perspective of one individual experiencing symptoms of disease we know that an optimistic diagnosis, a sense of a positive outcome can have a significant impact on their health. Indeed, in the absence of active medication i.e. when administering dummy pills, curative reactions often occur, this is in fact the 'placebo response' and such pills are called placebos.

Even in the absence of the placebo medication itself, i.e. when just this positive encouragement is given to patients and enables them to feel that they can do something about their situation, their survival and cure rates increase. This phenomenon was studied by David Spiegel at The University School of Medicine, California 1989 where he demonstrated that women with the **very late stage breast cancer doubled survival rate** when they took charge of their lives and used psychotherapy.

Indeed brain activity is known to release brain chemicals called neuropeptides; they are responsible for mediating sensory and emotional responses including hunger, thirst, pleasure and pain. The emotions were once thought to be a phenomenon of the brain; however these neuropeptides are released not only by the brain but by the nervous system all over the body. In addition we now know that they can be released by other organs, for example the digestive tract and adrenals, not only are we physically affected by our emotions but it appears that our whole body has the ability to store and express emotions. When you feel emotional this is not just your brain thinking your body is being affected, or your brain affecting your body, your body is physically affected by your emotions whether you think it or not.

> *"Through the millennia, humanity has more or less consciously known that all diseases ultimately have a psychic origin and it became a "scientific" asset firmly anchored in the inheritance of universal knowledge; it is only modern medicine that has turned our animated beings into a bag full of chemical formulas."*
>
> **Dr Ryke Geerd Hamer**

Dr. Candace Pert a graduate student in her mid-twenties discovered the 'opiate receptor', the cellular bonding site for endorphins, the body's natural painkillers. She was awarded her Ph.D. in pharmacology, with distinction, in 1974, from the Johns Hopkins University School of Medicine and conducted a National Institutes of Health (NIH) Postdoctoral Fellowship from 1974-1975. After 1975, she held a variety of research positions with the National Institutes of Health, and until 1987, served as Chief of Section, of Brain Biochemistry, Clinical Neuroscience Branch of the National Institute of Mental Health (NIMH).

In her book, *'Molecules of Emotion: The Science Behind Mind-Body Medicine'* Candace Pert explains:

> *"The tendency to ignore our emotions is "oldthink", a remnant of the <u>still-reigning paradigm</u> that keeps us focused on the*

*material level of health, the physicality of it. But the emotions
are a key element in self-care because they allow us to enter
into the bodymind's conversation. By getting in touch with our
emotions, both by listening to them and by directing them
through the psychosomatic network, we gain access to the
healing wisdom that is everyone's natural biological right."*

*"And how do we do this? First by acknowledging and claiming
all our feelings, not just the so-called positive ones. Anger,
grief, fear--these emotional experiences are not negative in
themselves; in fact, they are vital for our survival. We need
anger to define boundaries, grief to deal with our losses, and
fear to protect ourselves from danger. It's only when these
feelings are denied, so that they cannot be easily and rapidly
processed through the system and released, that the situation
becomes toxic...And the more we deny them, the greater the
ultimate toxicity, which often takes the form of an explosive
release of pent-up emotion. That's when emotion can be
damaging to both oneself and others, because its expression
becomes overwhelming, sometimes violent."*

**It appears that the problem is not so much in having negative
emotions but the judgement of those emotions, feeling that those
emotions are wrong or bad and therefore suppressing them.**

Just as we have demonstrated with the physical reactions of the body,
it is the suppression of these reactions that is most significantly
damaging. The parallels between the mind and body are outstanding;
suppressing emotions will have a potentially detrimental effect on the
body and consequently reflect in illness and susceptibility to disease.
Therefore emotional reactions are absolutely necessary to resolve the
emotional traumas and this affects the body as well as the mind.

Obviously emotional reactions themselves can be debilitating, if we do
not learn from our experiences and continue the trauma, we are of
course adding to our toxic load, however by suppressing the expression

of these reactions that would normally allow resolution, we could be compounding the situation further still.

Our perception of disease is in fact a double edged sword, not only do we have to deal with the trauma giving rise to the reaction, but if we are then to perceive the reaction itself as 'bad' we create additional trauma by the negative judgement of our responses. We grieve and then become upset with our upset, afraid and become afraid of being fearful, we suppress these feelings and we are now less able to deal with the trauma that caused the feeling in the first place.

Our focus on the reaction as being the problem once again obliterates the need to look at what we are reacting to, we are conditioned to suppress our so-called 'negative' emotions, if these reactions become too problematic then take a pill for your ill, convinced that there is something 'wrong' with you. Soon your ability to respond diminishes and your faith in your ability to heal and resolve will also decline. We spiral into a syndrome akin to the 'Nocebo' response.

13.2 The Nocebo Response

"Words are, of course, the most powerful drug used by mankind"

Rudyard Kipling

Various lines of research have shown how the pessimistic expectations of a patient, affects the physiology of the body, creating additional symptoms of disease. This is of course in complete contrast to the more well-known 'placebo response', where positive expectations affect the physiology in a positive manner, enabling patients to overcome disease.

Regarding the nocebo response, studies exist demonstrating significant changes in symptoms and the biochemistry of the body when patients are told they will be subjected to something harmful, Arthur Barsky, a psychiatrist at Boston's Brigham and Women's Hospital published a review in JAMA.;287(5):622-7. Feb 6 2002 and warned that:

> *"While the placebo effect refers to health benefits produced by a treatment that should have no effect, patients experiencing the nocebo effect experience the opposite. They presume the worst, health-wise, and that's just what they get."*

> **"They're convinced that something is going to go wrong, and it's a self-fulfilling prophecy**...*From a clinical point of view, this is by no means peripheral or irrelevant."*

A pertinent example of which can be found documented in the writings of Douglas Hume "Béchamp or Pasteur: A Lost Chapter in The History of Biology" regarding the issue of rabies and rabies vaccines. Here we see the difficulty in assessing the effect of medication if it is highly praised and subject to a large dose of placebo when compared to a disease diagnosis that creates fear and subject to an even larger dose of nocebo.

> *"The pity is that since Pasteur's day there should have been so much scare on the subject, for rabies is a complaint of the nerves and consequently fear is its primary factor. Various instances have been recorded of cases unquestionably brought on by suggestion. For example, two young Frenchman were bitten at Havre by the same dog in January 1853. One died from the effects, within a month, but before this, the other young man had sailed for America, where he lived for 15 years in total ignorance of the end of his former companion. In September 1868, he returned to France and heard of the tragedy and actually then himself developed symptoms and within three weeks was dead of rabies!"*

13.3 Learned Helplessness

Add this phenomenon to another trait of learned behaviour: Michelle Odent in his book 'Primal Health' looks at the impact of medical intervention, environment and social interaction on human development, from conception to first birthday. He quotes from experiments carried out by Martin Seligman in the 1960's:

> "They divided some dogs into two groups. The first group were given electric shocks from which they could do absolutely nothing to escape. The second group of dogs was placed in identical cages but given no shocks at all.
>
> The same two groups of dogs were then tested in a special box which had two compartments divided by a barrier. In one compartment, the dogs received an electric shock. But by jumping over a barrier they could escape the shocks. The second group of dogs, which had never had any electric shocks before, very quickly discovered the escape route and jumped over the barrier.
>
> But the astounding thing was that the first group of dogs – those which had previously been shocked – did not make any attempt to escape. They just crouched helplessly in the electric shock compartment. Even when the dogs were lifted over the barrier to the safe side, it still made no difference. They had learned from their first experience that nothing they did made any difference, and they were unable to control events. Seligman called this behaviour 'learned helplessness'"

Therefore what is the general impact of an approach to health care based on the perception of symptoms as mal-function and remedial action that encourages you to suppress these 'bad' reactions? Firstly we become convinced of the failings of the human body; the constant and pervasive message is that your symptoms are indicative of mal-function, therefore we are not motivated to remedy our situation through addressing causation but by suppressing symptoms and we quickly learn that there is nothing else that can be done; learned helplessness. Drug intervention leading to more intervention and ultimately for many, drug dependency. We are then motivated to health and disease interventions based on fear, fear of what will happen if we don't take the drugs, fear from the diagnosis itself with its concomitant nocebo response and its additional damaging effect on the human body. We become a helpless population whose fear is easily exploited, and easily manipulated by those that can take advantage of our fear, which, among other things, is the number one point of leverage in many commercial sales and none more so than pharmaceutical sales.

In order to summarise this section we will dissect an example of an illness and thereby illustrate the limitation in the orthodox approach mainly due to an absence of a body intelligence perspective.

So for example, suppose you have a heart condition such as angina, which manifests as pain in the heart created by a reduced blood flow to the heart muscle caused by a narrowing of the arteries. In the doctor's surgery or the pharmacy counter it is very uncommon indeed to address individual lifestyle issues to any degree; diet and lifestyle can predispose us to arterial damage, and the furring of the artery is often an attempt by the body to repair vascular damage.

However, you will be prescribed standard medication to widen the arteries and will often do nothing to address the root causes; many patients don't actually believe there is anything that could actually reverse the condition and are thereby well on their way to 'learnt helplessness'. You will be told of what can happen to you if your symptoms get worse, based on the many individuals in the orthodox medical system that do not attempt to resolve their underlying condition. These risks may not relate to you as an individual, but the possibility of that worst case scenario will form the basis of your treatment, this is your dose of nocebo. You will then be prescribed long-term medication with the concomitant fear of what can happen to you if all was to fail and go horribly wrong.

There is a complete line of research that is missing in the application of our Health Service: What predisposes us to make the arterial plaque (the material that is apparently clogging the arteries)? Are there physical as well as psychological factors? Does the arterial plaque have any function? What happens if I temporarily widen the arteries with medication but do not address the root causes, will my condition get worse? Even though the plaque contains cholesterol, is it simply the result of excess cholesterol in the diet? If we take drugs to suppress the body from producing cholesterol, does that address the cause and what of the implications of suppressing the formation of cholesterol; a necessary molecule of our body's biochemistry?

This line of research would have enabled us to find predisposing factors that cause the formation of plaque and to discover that the function of plaque, in the short-term, is to repair damaged blood vessels. Damaged in part by, free radicals, acid forming diet, dehydration, emotional trauma, and therefore pre-disposed by insufficient anti-oxidants, alkalising minerals, water and unresolved anxieties. This line of research and dissemination of information would have paved the way for knowledge of optimal lifestyle, which inevitably engages us with our relationship to our environment, lifestyle, nutrition and toxins, with the sense that there is something we can positively do to increase health and thereby reduce disease.

In order to take advantage of the body's innate ability to self-heal it is clear that we need to make a fundamental shift in the way we understand and deal with illnesses; a shift from the old mechanical orthodox model, (which has little understanding of the purpose and causes of symptoms), to a more holistic model which incorporates the detail and wider perspective of symptom purpose and causation.

CHAPTER 13 – SUMMARY

> The suppressing action of drugs will have detrimental effects on the body, but there are additional implications especially with regard to our psyche.

> The practise of suppressing symptoms comes from a belief system first, which is one that perceives symptom reactions as malfunctions and therefore bad for you.

> 'Believing' your symptoms to be bad induces fear and a reduced belief in your own abilities, thereby adding to the stress of the initial condition (nocebo).

> Promoting drug use instead of lifestyle adjustment induces a sense of helplessness and drug dependence (learnt helplessness).

> This desire to suppress also extends to emotional reactions which if suppressed can also affect mind and body detrimentally; emotions can be equally toxic if harboured in the body and left unresolved.

> Ultimately, the belief in suppression and the act of suppressing, induces, fear, helplessness and confusion which can in due course be disabling, disempowering and regressive.

CHAPTER FOURTEEN

14 Gaia - the way forward

The New Science of Immunology supports holistic medicine

The key issues when dealing with immune responses to microbial illnesses are:

> How to know and avoid disease conditions in the first place, what are the factors that contribute to disease and what role are microbes playing in our cellular function.

> How to provide a supportive environment for immune learning, without the need for immune crisis in the first place, given that environmental stimulus enables us to adapt and learn, i.e. how do we build a strong mind/body system to ensure immune success with the minimum of symptoms for our inevitable encounters with disease conditions?

> In the management of disease whilst in an immune crisis, how to treat the individual in order to resolve the acute illness quickly and successfully?

> What are the factors that contribute to immune failure and how do we reduce them and therefore how do we avoid chronic and invasive consequences?

> Lastly, given the unfortunate consequence of immune failure, chronic disease and inherited disease patterns, how do we address these chronic predispositions, i.e. the issues that have been unresolved in our own past and from previous generations?

We are beginning to understand the nature of immunity and realise that immune function is a whole body/mind process. In fact although we study the individual systems of the body and can understand the functions of various parts, the body/mind functions as a whole integrated system.

When you carry out any function, it is of course a whole body/mind process, for example you don't just eat with your digestive system but with all of your systems together, your digestive system, nervous system, endocrine system, cardio-vascular system, mental and emotional system; all of the systems are connected and are all necessarily involved.

Similarly you carry out immune function with all of the systems of the body, keeping out unwanted elements using all the mucous membranes of the body, eliminating using respiration, urination, perspiration, and defecation, coordinating using nervous and endocrine systems, supplying vital components with your digestive system, draining with the lymphatic system, responding also with mental and emotional system and so on.

Scientists are attempting to study immune function from a more integrated perspective, examining the effects of the mental and emotional state, together with the nervous system and immune system, this new discipline is called 'psychoneuroimmunology', here scientists conduct research into how these systems function as an integrated whole, and therefore what is the influence of the mind and nervous system on the classical immune system.

An international conference was held at the University of Perugia, in 1988 wherein thinkers and doers at the top of their fields (immunologists, biologists, ecologists, psychologists, philosophers) from all over the world, came to share their views on the new ways in which we envision the world, a new world of phenomena and dynamic interactions that cannot be modelled on the old mechanistic models. The purpose;

"...so that humanity can avoid the intense pain that is now coming from the misunderstanding of our planetary life".

The content of that meeting has been published in the book GAIA 2, the first held in California in 1981 considered Gaia as "a way of knowing". The Gaia hypothesis was first introduced in 1972 by James Lovelock and later co-authored with Lynn Margulis. Essentially the earth including the earth's environment, the content of the air, earth and water were to be considered an integral part of the life on earth, every element of the environment is influenced and produced by living systems. The earth is not simply an inanimate environment with living organisms exploiting its resources, but the environment itself would only exist in the form that it is because of life

...life and the environment have developed 'together'.

The waste products of one life form are used by another and elements that are needed by others are produced to varying degrees by other life forms, and there are of course very many life forms integrated within the earths soil, water and atmosphere, all contributing to each other, to the environment and equally responding to the environment. The earth's eco-system seems to mimic the eco-system of the human body, a micro-system reflective of the macro-system and responds in a similar manner to changes.

Notably when something appears in excess or some element changes, there are many systems that are able to utilise this excess which immediately feeds into other systems, such that the whole system maintains a high degree of equilibrium i.e. stability. Changes are responded to, such that there appears to be very little change in the overall levels, what Lovelock refers to as stable-self regulation, this self-regulation is an 'emergent' property of the whole. In the case of Gaia theory this can be elegantly demonstrated by creating models of the earth containing many organisms and adjusting parameters such as light, carbon dioxide and so on. The earth in conjunction with all its inhabitants behaves as though it were one individual, responding to these changes in order to maintain equilibrium, until the change is so great that a crisis occurs, from which point the equilibrium is disrupted usually to a new steady state.

This of course mirrors exactly the situation of an individual, responding to changes in the environment, maintaining stability until a point of crisis which we call an acute disease, a crisis that will culminate in a new steady state, one that we could learn from, be debilitated from or die from.

One of the contributors of Gaia 2, Francisco Varela discusses the nature of immunity from the point of view of immune learning and the more up to date concepts in life sciences and immunology. The evidence suggests that our immune system is of course tightly coupled to all of our systems and can recognise, learn and remember, it is not only involved in reacting to what is foreign but also involved in regulating the number of our own cells and beneficial micro-organisms.

> *'Our purpose here is to introduce a substantially different metaphor and conceptual framework for the study of immunity, one that puts the emphasis on the "cognitive" abilities of immune events'...*
>
> F. Varela

Immune responses are in fact similar to the learning processes that were previously assigned only to brain and nervous system function; this is the context in which F. Varela now observes and understands immune activity. Old metaphors of attack, defend, recognition and memory could not describe what we now know of immune activity; these newly acquired facts of immune activity gave rise to the term **Immu-knowledge**.

14.1 Immu-knowledge

Immunology contained simple mixed metaphors in trying to describe immune processes: Military; attack and defend, also recognition, learning and memory.

F. Varela Immu-knowledge in Gaia 2

The dominant model of our immune system.
Firstly in a militaristic model we identify the existence of an enemy, they are foreign and have the intention to harm us. They are therefore attacked and destroyed. Secondly this model suggests that our immune army is able to recognise the enemy and therefore would have to distinguish enemy from self.

It would be inconceivable to have all that information of all our possible enemies already on the inside, so these specialised cells and molecules must therefore be produced as, when, and if, needed. This learning would inevitably result in a cascade of destruction mediated by the immune system against the enemy, whilst avoiding our own cells; with the resulting memory of such an encounter, you would therefore be immune.

In this model, foreign molecules act as instructions to the immune system and the information is entirely directed from the outside. A 'playdough – style' learning, this theory, still held by many today, states that you can only be immune if you have had contact with the foreign agent and consequently could only be immune if you have had that disease.

However there were flaws with this and in fact this theory of immunity is only able to exist by ignoring the real issues:

The first problem is, if antibodies learn **only after** having been in contact with a foreign element by operating like a 'universal dough', it would be in contact with your own cells before it met a foreign element and therefore would have to know not to attack the self. In addition forming around an object like universal dough is not actual learning, otherwise the paper on which your signature is placed has 'learnt', it could be said to have an imprinted memory but not really learnt and with no ability to learn and problem solve as it were.

If the antibody is directed from the outside it would need to know what is foreign from what is not foreign BEFORE it met the foreign antigen.

Immu-knowledge… (Continued)

Therefore the idea of 'Tolerance' was introduced in 1900 by Ehrlich and here we are talking of tolerance to billions of types of our own molecules, cells, chemicals, foods, including viruses and bacteria that our immune system simply leaves alone because they are necessary for our functioning. Recognition would have to be more sophisticated than antibodies and lymphocytes acting like universal glue to non-self.

In addition immunologists have found that the antibody recognition is approximate, we have a repertoire of approximately 1020 antibodies which have to be able to recognise many more varieties of antigens that exist in the world. This ability of antibodies to recognise many different types of molecules in fact makes the problem even worse. This was partially solved with the theory of clonal selection, each lymphocyte produces its own type of antibody, one fits best and that lymphocyte reproduces and therefore genes are not changed but specific lymphocytes are selected for, not genetic but antigenic determination. (After-genetic determination).

The issue of self-recognition was not solved, however, self-recognition must mean that antibodies are able to recognise all possible self cells including those that are 'necessary non-self cells', without destroying them and each are able to recognise a variety of foreign antigens with the necessary destruction and elimination. The initial hypothesis was that antibodies have a range and the ones that do recognise the self are selected out, i.e. destroyed. Leaving only those that do not recognise the self and therefore only able to recognise foreign. So they are not distinguishing self, rather ONLY able to recognise a small range of foreign. This was thought to happen in the embryonic stages of development.

However it was later found that tolerance did develop over time and did not involve the destruction of lymphocyte clones. In addition lymphocytes themselves are not all formed during embryonic development and develop throughout later life. Also to destroy antibody clones that are capable of recognising self (because recognition is approximate) would delete huge chunks of lymphocytes severely compromising immune function.

These flaws in our immune theories have become more apparent as we discovered more about the immune system, which has lead to more useful theories of immunology that have been around since the 1970's, although many commercial scientists are finding it difficult to embrace these facts.

Immu-knowledge… (Continued)

Firstly we have discovered that **there are antibodies to self-cells** and even antibodies to antibodies, although not in the numbers that evoke destruction and elimination. Also animals that are not exposed to antigens from birth are able to develop full immune systems and **can react to antigens that they have never been exposed to before**. They are even capable of reacting to man-made chemical antigens that do not exist in the natural world.

Essentially in the natural world, we are exposed to small amounts of molecules in the food we eat and the air we breathe, we adjust to these through a network of immune cells that develop gradually. As do all biological networks; there appears to be an **ecosystem of antibodies and leukocytes adjusting <u>ALL</u> cell levels, molecules, particles – our own as well as foreign.**

So far from just eliminating foreign cells/molecules and leaving our cells alone we adjust to and adjust levels of all kinds of cells including our own, therefore there exists an interconnected system of reactions that continue all the time.

This is a positive task of self-assertion not a crisis motivated negative one. There are still reflex immune reactions that can occur when an antigen enters too quickly or in too large amounts and this has been the study of most of classical immunology.

The massive defensive responses are secondary characteristics, to say that immunity is fundamentally defence is as distorted as to say the brain is fundamentally about defence avoidance, we can do it but there's much more to brain activity, just as there is much more to immune activity. **When an immunologist injects large amounts of foreign material into somebody this evokes a response that appears to be externally instructed <u>but this is a highly contrived laboratory system.</u>**

14.1.1 Therefore "Know Thy Self"

These current observations and analysis of immune activity are of enormous significance. The immune system, it seems, develops normally in the absence of immune shocks because it is under constant challenge from the normal life processes of eating, breathing, moving, growing and just generally interacting with its environment. Furthermore it appears as though our own cells stimulate a small amount of immune activity creating a network of slightly charged immune cells that are constantly working and able to detect disturbances before greater problems arise.

> *"This is a positive task of self-assertion not a crisis motivated negative one."*

F Varela

The immune system acts like a sophisticated spider's web, it is able to know what is non-self because it knows what is self. Therefore the immune system does in fact react to itself and contrary to classical immunology the **immune system can react very strongly to elements it has never seen before.**

Because the immune system knows itself, it necessarily knows what is 'non-self'.

The suggestion is therefore that the immune system develops best by adjusting to *small disturbances*, as you would expect from the food and air that you take in, in fact such disturbances must also include all environmental disturbances, toxins, temperature, humidity, hydration, nutrition, emotions and so on. Any number of which could result in toxic overload, cell death and microbial imbalances. Immune reactions to unwanted elements are made through slight adjustments to the web of immune cells and antibodies that have been developing throughout life, therefore:

To have developed immunity, means to have 'learnt' to cope with your environment and therefore to be immune means to be able to deal with your environment.

We develop immune rashes so that we will able to eliminate blood poisons, the membranes of the body get stronger, inflammation becomes more efficient, we are more able to deal with separation, one step closer to independence and so on. As we learn to deal with those situations the appropriate systems develop and we become less likely to succumb to those issues later. We will in fact have more than one instance of what will be diagnosed as viral rashes, which are diagnoses by default; even measles itself will never be diagnosed by the detection of measles virus.

> *"Indeed, in the entire scientific literature there's not even one publication, where "viruses in the disease" the fulfilment of Koch's first postulate is even claimed. That means that there is no proof that from humans with certain diseases the viruses - which are held responsible for these diseases - have been isolated. Nevertheless, this is precisely what they publicly claim."*
>
> **Stefan Lanka**

We do in fact learn many things from conception to birth and adulthood; to breathe, regulate temperature, eat, walk, communicate, deal with the environment in a myriad of ways, all of which contributes to our learning which necessarily contributes to our immunity.

To suggest that we can be immune to one microbe and therefore immune to a disease because of the presence of an antibody to that microbe is exceptionally simplistic and consequently inaccurate. Additionally, to state that we can only be immune after having seen the microbe is demonstrably untrue. This puts the whole of vaccine theory into question; vaccines place microbial agents into the blood to give us a kind of forewarning as it was assumed that our strongest immune response happens only after having seen the pathogen at least once, this assumption has been proved wrong; we necessarily know what is 'non-self' (potential poisons and pathogenic microbes) because we know what is self.

This, of course, ties in with the observation that acute illnesses are more likely to happen in situations of increased stress, when a child is experiencing their developmental leaps and concomitantly separating from the parents; weaning off breast milk, accepting new foods, teething, learning to walk, learning to talk, potty training, starting nursery or new school, accepting a new sibling, parents going to work, and so on, these may also impact on dietary issues, changes in weather, increased toxins from food additives, insecticides and so on.

A vaccine or anti-microbial agent assumes that the microbe is the primary cause, which it is not, additionally a vaccine cannot hope to mimic a disease process, but only sensitises you to certain molecular elements and toxins in the vaccine. The purpose of the vaccine is to push your body into creating detectable levels of anti-bodies; the vaccine is not designed to stimulate a general immune response that enables you to deal with the real causations of disease. One danger is that vaccines trick the body into perceiving that its internal systems are being overrun by specific microbes, which over sensitise individuals to microbes that need to be kept in balance, therefore putting our bodies into red alert, and then with the use of additional pharmaceutical medication the medical profession suppresses subsequent immune responses.

Yes the immune system can mount defence mechanisms to toxic shocks, as would be the case in a full-blown illness, but the evidence points to the fact that for the development of immunity this is **neither necessary nor desirable**. Therefore, contrary to the immune theories of Jenner, you can be immune to illnesses that you have never had before and successfully cope with viruses and bacteria that you have never developed illnesses to, as is the case with most individuals that do not succumb to illnesses associated with the constantly evolving and changing bacteria and viruses that we are all exposed to.

Therefore immune systems learn as with other physical, mental and emotional learning, through trial & error and trial & success.

But learning only occurs if there is sufficient response to overcome the trauma. If there has been an initial failure, recurrent reactions constitute further trial & error until ultimately we experience success, which is why some people can have the so-called childhood illnesses more than once.

To understand the process of learning in one system, we can look at examples from any other human system, physically, mentally or emotionally. When learning to walk, it is <u>not</u> necessary for a child to fall from a great height in order to learn to balance. Learning appears to be maximised by exposure to <u>small</u> disturbances that through trial & error, enables success. Greater disturbances are in danger of creating a large degree of failure that subsequently compromises the individual so that they are now <u>less</u> able to succeed than they were before.

> *"And the trouble is, if you don't risk anything, you risk even more"*
>
> **Erica Jong**

In order to learn one cannot completely eliminate the risk of error, eliminate error and there is no learning, no possibility of error and you are in fact doing something you already know how to do. Once we are aware of the learning process we are able to minimise the consequences of error whilst also allowing the stimulus for learning. Vaccines appear to be mimicking a crisis in order to be 'immune' to that crisis; it would be like stimulating the reaction to getting run over by car as a necessary step in learning to cross the road. You would learn, but you may also consider it neither desirable nor necessary. The logical protection would be to teach your child road safety through small trial & error and trial & success lessons that do not involve your child actually getting hit by a car, so that they are able to <u>avoid</u> those great disturbances, i.e. able to avoid lorries, cars and buses, even those which they have never even seen before!

This suggests that immunity cannot be given to you as a drug any more than learning to walk can be given to you as a drug, drugs may help in a crisis but it is through your own response that you learn, in order for vaccines to stimulate immunity they would have to mimic very closely the stimulus to learning and our response would be a whole body/mind response that cannot simply be assessed by measuring levels of antibodies.

The question regarding the best way to gain health and immunity and therefore the best way to avoid serious disease hinges on the true nature of immune development, from childhood to adulthood. It is of course inextricably linked to every other area of development. Physically we have to learn to deal with increasing exposure to our environment, maintaining optimum levels of microbes, nutrients, temperature, and hydration, developing strong membranes, strong sense of self, adaptability and so on. This is all, of course, mirrored in our psyche, the child is learning to adapt, communicate, create boundaries, deal with the experience of separation, live independently and learn self-assertion.

There is no need to poison the blood of the body with vaccines to enhance immune responses, and eliminating germs by killing them doesn't address the susceptibility. We will get all the challenges we need through the normal processes of life. Remember a dangerous disease occurs in someone that is dangerously ill; they are overly stressed and/or under-resourced, the microbes are always there trying to help us out, they are responsible for nothing.

In reducing susceptibility to disease we need to adjust the parameters of our environment to promote optimum health, and stretch ourselves if we want to be able to deal with more adverse circumstances. It is vitally important to work with practitioners that understand the difference between suppression and expression of symptoms, and be prepared to adjust lifestyle where needed.

In acute diseases we are reacting to our environment and we have certain choices in treating disease, when for example we see a child with a nasal discharge and a cough, it is important to assess what the child is reacting to; what stress is the child under, how can we reduce the stress and how can we help the reaction. Is the child teething, moving from breast milk to a new food, starting nursery, reacting to an environmental trauma, previous trauma or expressing an inherited susceptibility? There are foods that add to phlegm and foods that help in the elimination, lifestyle adjustments that can reduce the stress, holistic therapies that help in the elimination of the catarrh, and therapies that can help in the resolution of inherited patterns.

14.2 Waning Vaccine Immunity

With the vaccine community promoting the idea that vaccines create immunity, they have to reconcile the fact that this so-called immunity is not 'life-long' as is natural immunity. We are therefore told that vaccine immunity wears off, which of course requires that we are given repeat doses of the vaccine. If we understand the nature of immune development and acknowledge the integration of our physiological systems together with mind and body we realise that immune development and consequently immunity, like learning to do anything, walking talking, eating etc, **cannot wear off**.

The only possibility of un-learning something is if we deteriorate so markedly in health that we become susceptible to ill-health generally, as is often the case in elderly, mal-nourished, severely traumatised etc. There can be no specific un-learning of one disease, **the reason vaccine immunity appears to wear off is that there was no immune learning in the first place.** When an individual develops a disease from which it was previously vaccinated this is because immunity has merely been delayed not because immunity has worn off.

With or without antibodies vaccinated individuals will succumb to those illnesses in the future if the issues of susceptibility come up later. Childhood illnesses occur later because the individual has had to overcome deeper problems before they could be healthy enough to express the childhood illness; these deeper problems are often exacerbated by the vaccine.

If a child has been forced to stop crying whilst experiencing an upset, then at some point in the future this upset may be expressed. The expression was however suppressed and the child has had to deal with the additional trauma of being made to feel wrong, bad, unsupported etc. If fortunate the child may eventually get to express the original upset, at this point there is no un-learning of any ability to deal with the trauma, it was never dealt with in the first place.

Rather than creating a waning immunity, vaccines delay immunity.

14.3 The way forward - a matter of addressing susceptibility

"The best time to plant a tree was 20 years ago. The second best time is now."

- Chinese Proverb

For some, we may appear to have painted a bleak picture and it would be easy to assume a state of powerlessness, victims of conspiracy, with feelings of guilt for what we should have done in the past. But the present way of the world, has obviously had to be that way, an integral part of the universal learning process. This could be equally positive as we may now see opportunities to resolve chronic disease and create health in ways that may have been obscured before.

CHAPTER 14 - SUMMARY

> ➢ 'Immune function' involves all of the systems of the body; even though we can separate the systems to observe and study the parts, ultimately we function as a whole.

> ➢ The immune system operates like all the physical, mental and emotional systems of the body and can 'learn'.

> ➢ Old metaphors such as 'attack and defend', 'self and non-self' are inaccurate representations of immune activity.

> ➢ The immune system learns through interaction with its environment and adapting to the small changes it encounters, such as in the food and air we take in.

> ➢ Learning through crisis, is possible though not necessary or desirable.

> ➢ The immune system knows what is foreign because it knows itself. Humans would recognise an alien from outer space as being 'different' because we know what humans look like.

> ➢ The idea that we need to inject foreign proteins in the form of vaccines to enable immune learning is based on outdated immunology.

> ➢ Historically immunologists have studied crisis reactions in contrived laboratory situations which are not reflective of real life immune function.

> ➢ Although the pharmaceutical industry uses very update and cutting edge technologies, its approach to immune treatments and vaccines are based on old theories of immunology.

> ➢ Immune learning and immune building is much easier than we have been lead to believe.

CHAPTER FIFTEEN

15 How re-framing disease can help remove fear, avoid poor treatment choices and improve health naturally.

"The processes of disease aim not at the destruction of life, but the saving of it."

Frederick Treves, 1905

15.1 Principles of Immune Reactions & 'Infectious' Disease

Historically the immune system was simply thought of as a specialised group of cells designed to defend the body against attacking microbes. The groups of cells given the most importance regarding immune function were thought to reside in the blood and were capable of producing antibodies.

The microbe was thought to cause the disease by infecting the individual and having seen a particular microbe once, the immune system could somehow memorise their form. This immune memory could only be obtained by exposure to that specific pathogen, once memorised, the immune system, in any subsequent attacks, could more easily render microbes harmless and this ability to remember the microbe was thought to be due to the action of antibodies.

We now realise that this oversimplification is flawed in two very important aspects, <u>firstly</u> in relation to our understanding of infectious disease and <u>secondly</u> in our understanding of the immune system.

1. Regarding infectious disease, from the time of the popularisation of germ theory with Pasteur (1860s), scientists from Béchamp in the 1850's to those of the present day, have demonstrated that microbes are the <u>result</u> of nutritional changes, hormonal changes, toxins and physically damaged tissue within the body, and that microbes that are always present, will change in number and type according to the environment of the body. Pasteur on his death bed quoted by his old friend, Professor Renon, who attended him in his final illness:

   "Bernard was right. **The germ is nothing. The soil is everything.**"

   Consequently, trying to kill microbes, without addressing the reasons for their proliferation, is ultimately futile and will lead to recurrent problems, including the problems associated with the side effects of the drug. Microbes can be transferred from one person to another but without an existing susceptibility there is no disease. Epidemic diseases affecting groups of individuals at one time are reflective of; common susceptibilities within common inheritance, common conditions of nutrition, common weather patterns, common pollutants, common emotional stresses and so on. In addition, the action of the microbe itself is entirely dependent on where the microbe is in the body and therefore an illness cannot simply be caused by the infection of a microbe and the disease cannot be defined by the presence of a microbe, as most microbes that are said to cause serious diseases are present in all of us.

2. The immune system itself is involved in the elimination of toxins and maintaining microbes in a symbiotic relationship with our internal systems, an integral part of which are the mucous

membranes separating the internal blood system and organs from the external environment. The environment surrounding the membranes of: the skin, urinary, respiratory and digestive tracts will vary according to its location and essential to the functioning of many of these membranes are the microbes that live there.

As we have mentioned previously, there are many more microbes in your body than your own cells. The functioning of the immune system is actually dependent on these microbes, so, far from being a simple attack and defence issue, the immune system has the job of balancing these components within the various parts of the body, as they are in fact part of your immune system. Antibodies are also just a very small part of the immune system involved in balancing our own cells and foreign cells; they do not operate by attacking foreign elements and leaving our own cells alone. We also know that memory capabilities are a function of many tissues of the body and not just antibodies. Also antibodies require the cooperation of other cells to complete a successful immune response; a more significant immune role appears to be in the function of the other immune cells that do not produce antibodies. In addition immune function is enhanced through successful detoxification and elimination processes not the mere presence of antibodies. It appears that the vast numbers of antibodies measurable after vaccines is a contrived experimental situation and reflects extreme trauma wherein antibodies function as a last resort.

15.2 A Re-Classification of Infectious Illness

Currently many so-called infectious illnesses are classified according to the microbe that is thought to be responsible for the illness: measles, mumps, polio etc.

This has various drawbacks:

> The concept of an infectious illness and classification based on the microbe gives the impression that the microbe has somehow entered the system and caused the illness, when in fact the microbe would probably have been there all along.

> The presence of the microbe implies the presence of illness when in fact most people have these microbes and have no symptoms of disease.

> In individuals with a so-called infectious disease there are many other microbes present and many other disease factors present that can also be implicated in the disease, yet we choose one microbe and classify the illness according to that.

> Many different microbes are associated with the same illness, but these illnesses will have to be classified by a different name according to the presence of the other microbe, even though all other elements and symptoms of the disease are identical, e.g. meningitis and septicaemia from meningococcal B or meningococcal C or Haemophilus Influenza B.

> Classifying the disease according to the microbe is even more problematic when we consider that one microbe can be associated with many different kinds of illnesses.

Therefore if we turn our attention to the patient, a classification of illness according to the patient reaction <u>as well as</u> the type of microbes present, may create a more accurate picture of the pathology.

The <u>nature</u> of an infectious illnesses or rather what we shall now term a microbial illness will therefore depend on the following:

1. <u>The Patients Level of Immune Development</u>, how much of the immune system has developed and how much of the present illness is concerned with immune development - this is usually a function of age.

2. <u>The Amount of Toxicity Within the Patient</u>, how much toxicity is present in the body and how far has it penetrated into the

patient, i.e. into which systems of the body; digestive tract, blood, nervous system, etc.

3. <u>The susceptibility of the patient</u>, at what level does the patient operate, what stage of miasm i.e. how is the individual predisposed to react as a result of previous successes or failures, inherited or acquired.

Taking each issue in turn we are therefore able to classify microbial illnesses into one of three types each with a preponderance of one of the above factors.

1. **Developmental illnesses** – a function of immune development.

2. **Environmental illnesses** – relates mainly to toxicity and environmental stress.

3. **Immune deficient illnesses** – a function of reduced reactive ability.

There will of course be some overlap with certain illnesses and given the dynamic nature of human responses we will also demonstrate how illnesses can start off as one type but then develop into another, according to susceptibility, environment and disease management.

15.2.1 Developmental illness

These include some of what are classically known as the childhood illnesses, as we elaborate on the nature of these responses we shall see that they can equally occur in adulthood.

For the purposes of medical study the body has been divided into separate systems, each classified according to its main function, for example; the digestive system, endocrine system, nervous system, cardio-vascular system, respiratory system, immune system etc. In looking at the developmental illnesses (childhood illnesses), much of our efforts are focused on the immune system, in terms of function and development. However the body doesn't function using single systems and there are no distinct lines where one system starts and another finishes.

For example in dealing with poisons and associated microbes in the digestive tract, all systems have an integrated function; the digestive system plays a part in creating boundaries using the intestinal membrane, enzymes from the liver, pancreas and intestinal mucosal wall will help to break down certain molecules, resident microbes limit the growth of disease associated microbes, the blood and cardio-vascular system bring white blood cells to appropriate areas; hormones of the endocrine system regulate blood pressure, vasodilation and permeability; kidneys of the genitourinary system filter the blood; the nerves of the nervous system coordinate voluntary and involuntary muscle movement and so on.

Therefore, when considering immune development, there will be a concomitant development of other systems, including mental and emotional behaviour; each system is in fact inextricably linked to other systems.

We shall at first consider the mucous membranes of the human body. In the digestive tract this is therefore part of the digestive system, but also the immune system, endocrine system, nervous system, it has elimination functions as well as absorption and assimilation functions. This membrane provides, among other things, an effective barrier between the external environment and our internal systems (blood, organs and nervous tissue). A new-born child does not have a fully developed immune system, including therefore underdeveloped membranes; these are more porous than in a healthy adult with fewer resident microbes. Similarly many detoxifying enzymes and immune cells have not yet developed, kidney and liver function is also minimal.

Consequently in order to carry out digestion functions, foods have to be simple; hence the necessity for breast milk or similar food, (more complex foods could not be broken down and would actually cross the delicate membranes of the digestive system and poison the child). Similarly exposure to other potential toxins in the environment would have more severe consequences in a child than an adult – smoke, cosmetics, pharmaceutical drugs, alcohol, chemical additives, pollutants etc; the new-born child is less able to keep things out and less able to detoxify poisonous elements once within their system.

Remember, any acute reaction can be brought about by a combination of factors:
1. An increased amount of toxicity
2. Any physical or emotional stress that could adversely affect the system
3. Immune suppression

Most of the toxicity for the average child comes from what enters the digestive tract (ignoring the effects of drugs and vaccines) and as previously discussed, should there be anything in the diet that the child is unable to cope with then the child will react by eliminating. In the first instance this could be mucus elimination (nasal discharge, cough), vomiting and diarrhoea, (an inflammatory response cannot be produced in the first days, this ability takes some time to develop).

One of the most significant emotional stresses experienced by a child involves separation, mainly from the mother. In fact, the development of a child is intimately bound to the development of an independent self, with an ability to function without the parents, with strong discerning boundaries able to keep out what is detrimental for them and allow in what is needed. There are therefore strong parallels with both physical and psychological development.

Consequently the developmental milestones of, for example, teething, weaning, walking, talking, etc will take a child closer to independence but simultaneously further away from mother. There is therefore an accompanying stress associated with these events, allied to a certain amount of frustration that accompanies any learning or breakthrough process. It is therefore no coincidence that illnesses often occur at these points in a child's life. At these times of most stress, immune function is weaker and therefore toxins can build up with the accompanying accumulation of microbes.

Exposure to toxins, as described in the previous chapters, could lead to a build-up of toxicity that could cross the membranes into the blood with the accumulation of viruses. The elimination of this, involves blood immune cells and the phenomena of viral shedding i.e. "the rash", as in measles, rubella, chickenpox and the numerous rashes of children that are now classified as "just a virus".

The resolution of the blood toxicity by this elimination leads to a more integrated robust membrane, more able to keep out toxins and microbes from the blood i.e. 'natural immunity', as you would gain from naturally contracting measles. Suppression of this process, would lead to a build-up of toxins within the blood, a more leaky membrane and consequently the child would be sensitised to elements that can more easily gain access to the blood system and may be left with symptoms of 'allergies'. (See previous section on allergies).

Orthodox paediatricians, alternative health practitioners and parents, have noticed that after childhood illnesses there is often a developmental leap in the child, this is because the illness often occurs at the point of learning. The learning can involve any issue but will always involve many systems at once; learning to digest new foods, learning to produce new enzymes, learning to eliminate certain blood poisons, learning to create a fever, learning to produce certain immune reactions, weaning off of breast milk, teething, learning to crawl, walk, talk, all of which may also be accompanied by the stress of separation and with the difficulties and frustrations of the learning process itself.

The illness is an attempt to resolve an underlying issue, the issue will be different in different individuals, if an issue isn't there, the illness itself cannot resolve it: Two children fall and bruise their knees, one is learning to ride a bike, one learning to ice skate, resolve the issue, heal the bruising and one child is one step closer to learning to ride a bike and the other to ice skate. The specific bruising is not a pre-requisite for either and obviously the resolution of bruising in a child that is not learning to skate or ride will <u>not</u> result in a child that is able to ice skate or able to ride a bike.

> *"Doctor, will I be able to play the piano after my broken arm has healed?"..."Of course" says the doctor..."Great" says the patient, having never played the piano before.*

All illnesses are unique to the individual issues of each patient; the manifestation of the same illness may be as a result of a variety of different learning issues. The symptoms of measles, for example, are the end result of a process that started some time before. After measles, one child is more able to talk, another more able to balance, another more able to digest new foods, or deal with emotional stress.

But similar issues may also be occurring at the same time as other patients by virtue of their similar learning process and environment; children of a similar age, learning similar things, experiencing similar frustrations, in a similar environment could have similar reactions. Their illnesses are NOT simply by virtue of being in the presence of the same 'bug', otherwise all people exposed to that 'bug' would have that illness and they don't.

The disease measles for example is the infiltration and build-up of blood poisons in a child with an immune system that is not yet capable of an efficient inflammatory response, with relatively weak membranes and at a point of crisis, often when they are most stressed, physically, toxically, mentally or emotionally. Resolve the crisis, eliminate the poisons and many systems have learnt, leaving the child less susceptible to those issues after.

Similarly you do not 'need' a specific illness for a specific development to take place, any more than you need to break a leg in order to learn how to ride a bike. The public perception that 'there isn't so much measles around' is reflective of the perception that the disease can only be caused by one specific bug that we can get rid of. However if the incidence of measles (and essentially measles-like illnesses) diminishes, this means that many individuals are either not reaching that point of crisis and are not resolving their issues in that way (just as there are children who learn to ride a bike without breaking their legs) or they may not be healthy enough to produce skin reactions that resolve in that manner.

However you cannot learn to ride a bike without ever falling off and so as with immune development, it is inherently 'a learning process', which necessarily involves 'trial & error' and 'trial & success', the extent and exact manifestation of the error, is dependent on the individual. If your child becomes blood toxic at a point where immune development is occurring then they will develop symptoms of measles or immune rashes regardless of whether someone else has it or not. Remember the example of a country like Australia with good disease notification, it is noted that children develop childhood illnesses even though isolated from others for months, therefore whether 'it' is around or not.

But children could equally learn without the obvious manifestation of a crisis reaction, i.e. without the inflammatory skin rash, just as children learn to walk and ride without the crisis of broken bones. Minimising the consequences of our learning mistakes will therefore be important, reducing the toxic load on the child, minimising physical and emotional stress, etc. but eradicating the error from the process of trial & error and trial & success is not possible.

In order that we minimise the consequences of error, we therefore need to understand the issues inherent in the disease process, what is the human body reacting to in symptoms of dis-ease? In the developmental illnesses of children, these will be, for example; separation issues, the rate at which they are learning to gain independence, the amount of time away from parents, learning to walk, talk, weaning, new foods, toilet training, dealing with toxins in food, pollutants in their air, on their skin, in their environment, emotional stresses of the family environment. If your child is ill, these are the stresses that will need to be reduced, in fact, as everyone is probably aware, when their child is unwell and if the illness is not properly resolved, there is often a period of regression where they become more dependent and they naturally reduce the developmental demands on themselves.

Here you will understand how groups of children in similar stresses will succumb to similar illnesses, and how childhood illnesses suddenly appear even in isolated families and communities where they could not have just been transferred from an outside person with the same illness.

So we see there is a striking correlation between illness and weather change, change of seasons, a correlation between illness and childhood separation (i.e. starting nursery, school or university, a new sibling, their favourite teacher leaving), common environmental poisons in food, water and the air we breathe, common family stresses, fear of illness, divorce, death or fear of death of a family member, loss of employment by the main provider etc, the microbes were always present but now the patients susceptibility changes and we see symptoms of illness in an individual or similar group.

If we remember our discussion of inherited patterns of illness we also know that the susceptibility of the child will be determined by the inherited patterns of the parents (the inherited miasm). This may therefore predispose a child to:

- ➤ Skin illnesses – measles, rubella, chicken pox, etc or
- ➤ Glandular illnesses – tonsillitis, quinsy, inflamed adenoids, appendicitis
- ➤ Lung conditions – croup, bronchitis, whooping cough etc.

Which therefore influences the kinds of microbial illnesses that manifest in the child; the microbial illness cannot therefore be caught but develops if the susceptibility exists within the child. This is why most children in contact with other children with a so-called infectious illness do not contract the illness. Remember the classification of a polio epidemic is of the order of 35 in 100,000, and other illnesses are less than that.

It is interesting to note that when a child goes to nursery for the first time they are often prone to green nasal discharges, coughs and colds. From the old germ theory perspective it is often commented ...that these colds are caused by 'picking up bugs from the nursery'. On closer examination we can see the incongruence in this:

From a germ theory perspective we are lead to believe that children step into nurseries where the inhabitants have been cultivating bugs... bugs that have little access to the outside world, that have not come in contact with these children before and therefore can only be caught within the confines of the nursery building. Which, obviously, does not make sense, these microbes are present everywhere, on the child, in the child, in its environment, home, food etc.

Why do so many children succumb to these illnesses at the same time? This is due to the similarity in susceptibility as a consequence of the similarity of the individuals exposed to similar conditions at the same time... that is, children of a similar age group that are learning to be without their parents, often for the first time, learning to walk at similar times, toilet training at similar times and so on. The spread of disease usually follows an age group even though they are in contact with other age groups, or follows siblings with similar miasmatic (inherited) susceptibilities and/or similar home stresses and nutritional conditions. Given that the microbe is always present, if we are to understand microbial illnesses we need to understand the conditions that support them, trying to detect where the microbes come from will invariably lead you back to the patient.

Interestingly one common homeopathic medicine that will often remedy that state of the nursery school child with green discharge, is a remedy called pulsatilla and this remedy is used to help someone when they are feeling emotionally abandoned. Once this is resolved in the child, the mucus symptoms are similarly resolved. Resolution occurs when the child no longer suffers the consequences of being left and able to enjoy life in the absence of parents with the faith that their parents will return. The condition is a product of the susceptibility of the child and not due to attacking microbes that lurk within the confines of nursery buildings. Because of course, these microbes have always been present within the child.

Epidemics can give the impression that 'a bug is spreading around', however the actual spread and incidence of disease would suggest otherwise. In epidemic situations the onset of the disease will occur in individuals in many different places that are separated by 100's of miles, mountains, valleys, in different cities etc and will instantaneously start at the same time. This would suggest that there is a mass susceptibility that is caused by the conditions that are applicable to large areas at the same time. If disease were primarily caused by microbes without the necessary susceptibility, epidemics would follow a domino effect by person to person transfer, or at the very least airborne transfer, at a rate that would be limited by the speed at which the microbe could get from one person to another. Analysis of disease spread suggests that this is not the case. Flu viruses ever present, constantly changing, follow distinct epidemics according to weather change and environmental influences they happen instantaneously over very large distances in the minority of the population.

The consequences of what you do depend where you are. Add water to a thirsty plant and you may save it - add to a water-logged plant, and you may kill it.

We can appreciate that acute illnesses of childhood can therefore resolve inherited patterns from their parents; conversely, unresolved illnesses will add to the chronic patterns that already exist within the child. From the observation of these illness patterns it is possible to chart the progression of chronic illness in both their physical and emotional manifestations.

We see that the first kinds of illness involve the skin, with irritation, fears and insecurities, hunger at night, fear of the dark etc, part of what homeopaths have classified as the 'psoric miasm', if these are unresolved then deeper chronic illnesses affect the glands and lungs with coughs, a desire and sensitivity to milk, discontentment and tantrums. This deeper pattern of illness homeopaths have classified as the 'tubercular miasm'; there are further stages of chronic disease patterns that eventually lead to one of the lower levels involving - cancer, the 'carcinosin miasm', with lack of assertion, loss of identity, obsessions, deep fears, martyrdom and malignancies.

Revisiting Jenner

If we revisit the period of Edward Jenner, we are told that he experimented with a boy called James Phipps, and gave him the first vaccine, produced from the pustules of cowpox. If the boy James Phipps had resolved this blood poisoning we may have expected the manifestation of some kind of eliminatory rash. This did not occur, so was he left with an unresolved condition or had it been resolved in a manner that may not have been noticed or recorded? From our earlier text we have noted:

> James Phipps was declared immune to smallpox but died of tuberculosis at the age of 20. Convinced of the virtue of vaccination Edward Jenner inoculated his 18-month-old son with swinepox, on November 1791 and again in April 1798 with cowpox, he too died of tuberculosis at the age of 21.

Having a more holistic understanding of disease, being knowledgeable of the nature of unresolved illness, knowing the consequences of immune failure and deeper chronic disease, Edward Jenner would have known that both James Phipps and his son died of what we know in homeopathy as the deeper miasmatic 'tubercular disease'. They did not develop the rash of smallpox, but in this instance, due to the nature of the blood poisoning induced by the vaccination procedure, they subsequently developed tuberculosis, their disease was in fact driven deeper, and far from being immunised they were in fact immune compromised.

It is therefore predictable that if chronic disease is not resolved then we move deeper into the miasms and with the modern day use of childhood vaccination and widespread use of immune suppressive medication, we can see that this is in fact happening. It is therefore apparent that this deterioration to the lowest levels of health may in fact take generations and so the effects of vaccines and suppression are more apparent in children that have immune compromised parents. This is why there is a higher incidence of autism in children with parents that have immune sensitivities, why vaccine damage is more likely in children whose parents have immune sensitivities and why something as harmful as mercury will create more problems in individuals with a history of immune sensitivities.

One of the low stage chronic disease patterns is called the carcinosin miasm; the patterns are observable signs and symptoms and are not based on any prior theory. Individuals in the carcinosin miasm show symptoms and characteristics of poor assertion, poor boundaries, are unable to assert their desires, easily pushed into doing what they don't want to do, often doing for others to the detriment of themselves, they appear nice, they feel guilty when attending to their own needs, they are overly attached to others, overly attached to their mother, have difficulties with boundaries and attachment issues to their own children, fearful when taking responsibility, easily coerced by fear, a history of no childhood illness, history of difficulty weaning from the breast or in fact no breast milk, often sensitive to environment and foods, their illnesses become invasive, they do not overcome acute illnesses easily if at all, they have a tendency to tumours and malignancies, difficulties with fertility and being able to have their own children.

The characteristic pattern of signs and symptoms of individuals of the carcinosin miasm are in fact the opposite of what we are trying to develop in our children. From foetal development to an adult we are wanting to create a nurturing environment that in fact takes our children to a place of independence, where the individual has a strong sense of self, strong boundaries, able to allow in what is beneficial and keep out what is detrimental, feed themselves, assimilate a wide variety of foods, with a digestive system that can keep out what is harmful and allow in what is beneficial, able to talk for themselves, to know what is their issue from what is someone else's, feel able to attend to their own needs and able to choose when to attend to the needs of others. What in fact may be described as successful adaptation to the environment, in the wider context these are the characteristics of true immunity.

Clearly the passage of time from child to adult is not just an issue of size; ideally children are not just bigger foetuses and adults are not just bigger children.

One of the ways we have been able to confirm the presence of a chronic miasm when the symptoms are barely manifest is by using the associated remedy to see if the patient responds. The carcinosin remedy has often been used to good effect after a child has suffered the effects of vaccination, confirming the carcinosin susceptibility of the child; in fact carcinosin has become the most common childhood remedy because of the use of vaccination, and immune suppression in general

Interestingly, as noted in a previous chapter regarding the measles rash, orthodox experiments also confirm that suppression predisposes individuals to cancer. The Lancet Jan 5th 1985:

> ...It was known that, some did not produce the typical measles rash: In adulthood, (average age in the study was 38 years), for those with antibodies but NO rash, there was shown to be an increased incidence of immunoreactive diseases, sebaceous skin diseases, degenerative diseases of bone and cartilage, and certain tumours.

The report concludes that, at the time of infection, it may be dangerous to interfere with the immune response by administering a passive immunisation to suppress the rash. It also states... "The absence of a rash may imply that intracellular virus *(poisons)* escapes neutralisation during the acute infection and this, in turn, might give rise to the development of diseases subsequently". (My italics).

The use of suppressive medication is in fact suppressing the development of the immune system and of course other systems; it is practised without an understanding of the underlying developmental issues. With immune suppression, we are stopping the attempts of the body to resolve these apparently physical issues, and consequently in a subtle, pervasive and now very extensive manner we are inhibiting physiological and psychological development. Physical boundaries do not develop and the concomitant psychological behaviour is similarly impeded.

Using the insights of above, we can see that vaccines penetrate the boundaries of the human being; deliver a cocktail of harmful substances and any subsequent attempts at elimination is being suppressed. We are forcing our children to accept what is physiologically and psychologically harmful at a time when they are least able to cope, it is of no surprise therefore to learn that we are creating syndromes of the carcinosin miasm, individuals with poor boundaries, poor assertion, sensitised and lacking independence.

As the level of chronic disease deepens in our children then of course the ability to produce healthy skin reactions is lost, a child in a deep carcinosin chronic will have to move up through several levels before they are capable of the typical measles rash. For example we now see the phenomena of atypical measles in children, teenagers and adults, the medical definition being:

> An altered expression of measles, atypical measles begins suddenly with high fever, headache, cough, and abdominal pain. The rash may appear 1 to 2 days later, often beginning (in contrast to typical measles) on the lower limbs spreading towards the centre of the body. Swelling (oedema) of the hands and feet may occur. Pneumonia is common and may persist for 3 months or more, occasionally with enlarged spleen and liver.

Atypical measles is not allied to different poisons and different viruses, it is the same blood trauma wherein the same measles viruses can be found as experienced in children with typical measles, however the responses of the patients are more severe and the symptoms last longer. Atypical measles is a product of 'atypical patients' i.e. often in older children and adults that have not yet carried out the immune development that many (more typical patients) do at a younger age, characteristically as defined in medical text books it occurs in vaccinated individuals. **Measles in older children is <u>not</u> because it wasn't around for them to catch when they were younger.**

These individuals have a deeper miasmatic susceptibility, they are unable to eliminate blood poisons efficiently through the normal skin rash; other organs are affected and the elimination process itself less efficient. Consequently these developmental illnesses occur later in adulthood for some, but may never occur for others. The reduced incidence of measles in children and increased incidence of allergies and autoimmune disease is indicative of deteriorating health not increasing health and has nothing to do with measles being around or not being around.

This does not mean that a child without a history of measles is necessarily unhealthy, there are many subtle ways of immune learning that will not appear as the typical illness, some are also too mild to distinguish and this is also a sign of good health. So the absence of apparent childhood illness can be indicative of good health, but if associated with illnesses from the lower miasms will be indicative of poor health.

The typical childhood illness that culminates in the viral rash will serve to:

> Eliminate toxins, cell debris and viruses from the blood, allow the development of the immune system and other associated systems in the child, enhance the development of the mucous membranes and skin; make it harder for toxic and microbial elements to gain access to the internal systems of the body, create immunity to many kinds of illnesses, resolve emotional traumas in the child (often separation), resolve inherited physical and emotional susceptibilities from the parents and liberate energy for other developmental issues that are currently taking place.

It is very naive to think of a childhood illness as simply an illness caused by a microbe attacking the human body; consequently the practice of vaccination does not mimic the illness process at all. The level of toxicity introduced into the child is far greater than would happen when contracting the illness naturally, the mode of toxin accumulation by injecting under the skin is not the mode in which these illnesses manifest naturally, the age when these toxins are introduced by the use of vaccination, does not occur at an age when the child is necessarily ready to learn that process, (we are all at different stages of development), and finally the elimination process that culminates in immunity very rarely happens and when it does it is usually suppressed by the use of pharmaceutical drugs of which Calpol (anti-fever medication) is the number one offender.

15.2.2 Environmental Illness

This group of illnesses are due mainly to toxicity and they can occur in individuals with fully developed immune systems as well as in children with under-developed immune systems, they include illnesses such as cholera, typhoid, and hepatitis. When the individual has sufficient toxicity to support the microbe, then the illness is the crisis point at which the body will try to eliminate. If the individual resolves the toxic state and adjusts lifestyle accordingly then recurrences do not occur, if however they continue to subject themselves to these conditions then recurrences do occur.

Immunity from the microbe itself exists in individuals that are not sufficiently toxic to allow the microbe to proliferate, but immunity from the microbe does not exist if the conditions that cause their proliferation persist. For example cholera is an illness characterised by vomiting, diarrhoea, fever, sweating, malaise etc, symptoms may vary according to the individual, this symptom reaction is as a result of toxicity within the digestive system, usually from dirty water, it is simply not due to the presence of the microbe as many people have it but show no symptoms. However this is not immunity, as we would see in the case of childhood illnesses. Epidemiological evidence shows that as soon as toxic drinking water conditions exist, then cholera symptoms return.

For many years a cholera vaccine was promoted and given to individuals in epidemic situations as a preventative, however this is no longer given because the authorities (The World Health Organisation) now admit that the vaccine does not work and confirm that unless clean water and hygienic practice is in place then cholera will persist and the vaccine will not stop the spread of the disease.

Note that hygiene refers to cleanliness and appropriate waste disposal, not to be confused with aseptic, which refers to the absence of microbes. Hygienic = the elimination of the toxins that support pathogenic microbes.

Hepatitis means inflammation of the liver, the liver is the main organ of detoxification in the human body, almost all food that enters the digestive system, once absorbed into the blood, is taken to the liver to be processed and detoxified accordingly. Hepatitis occurs in individuals that have overly burdened their liver; consequently the illness occurs in certain high risk groups; alcohol users, drug users, people that undergo blood/plasma transfusions, those that are malnourished and with unclean dietary habits.

At first one virus was found and the illness was labelled according to the virus, interestingly now at least 5 different viruses have been found from Hep A to E with their various sub-groups. Such illnesses are a direct result of toxic conditions imposed on the liver, the presence of the virus could equally be as a result of toxicity as opposed to the cause of the liver damage. Any one virus can be present and symptoms can vary from minimal to lethal, and therefore the severity of the illness is a function of the susceptibility i.e. state of the host not a function of the virus.

At this juncture it is surely interesting to quote Florence Nightingale once again:

Florence Nightingale...

"Is it not living in a continual mistake to look upon disease as we do now, as separate entities which must exist, like cats and dogs, instead of looking upon them as the reactions of kindly nature against the conditions which we have placed ourselves?

I was brought up by scientific men to believe that smallpox was a thing of which there was once a specimen in the world, which went on propagating itself in a perpetual chain of descent, just as much as there was a first dog or pair of dogs, and that smallpox would not begin itself any more than a new dog would begin without there having been a parent dog.

Since then I have seen with my eyes and smelt with my nose smallpox growing up in first specimens, either in closed rooms or overcrowded wards where it could not by any possibility have been "caught" but must have begun. Nay, more, I have seen diseases begin, grow and pass into one another. Now dogs do not pass into cats. I have seen for instance, with a little overcrowding, continued fever grow up, and with a little more, typhoid fever, and with little more, typhus, and all in the same ward or hut.

For diseases, as all experience shows, are adjectives not noun substances. The specific disease doctrine is the grand refuge of weak, uncultured, unstable minds, such as now rule in the medical profession. There are no specific diseases, there are only specific disease conditions."

With such illnesses, from a disease management point of view, it is imperative to support the body with, re-hydration, nutritional supplementation where appropriate and therapeutic interventions that aid the dis-ease response. Many people do die when conditions are severe and their constitutions are weak, but those that die are not associated with more deadly microbes than those that survive, the microbes are the same as in those individuals that easily recover. However, in severe cases the patients are more toxic and are weaker, suppression of the elimination attempts of the body may in fact worsen the condition and can lead to invasive consequences, which brings us to section 3.

15.2.3 Immune deficient

This class of illnesses may also be described as the invasive infections; paralytic poliomyelitis, meningitis, encephalitis, septicaemia: they are due to toxins and microbial proliferation within the interior of the body i.e. beyond the membranes of the digestive tract, lungs, skin etc, and no longer secured within the lymphatics, joints, fat cells, liver etc they can therefore affect the nervous system.

Here we see that toxins and microbes have access to the other organs, nerves, meninges and brain tissue and is a consequence of the failure to keep this toxicity and the corresponding microbes out of the internal tissues of the body. The microbes themselves do not have to be caught from anywhere, as they are commonly part of the natural microbes that inhabit the body, usually in the external tracts of the digestive system, respiratory system, genitourinary system and the skin. This is a fact that often comes as a great surprise to members of the general public AND many health professionals. Polio, Hib, E.Coli, Meningococcal B, C, etc all microbes that are normally present within the tracts of the respiratory and digestive systems of everyone.

What enables them to *apparently* cause such devastating illnesses in a very small percentage of people but not in the vast majority of others? The polio example is immeasurably instructive when considering the issues of invasive consequences and the phenomenon of vaccination.

Polio (paralytic poliomyelitis) was in fact a disease of the developed world USA Europe and Australia. The illness had been described earlier in the 1900's and researchers found that nerve poisons entering the food chain caused the symptoms of acute flaccid paralysis or infantile paralysis. It later reached epidemic proportions (20-35 in 100,000) in the 1950's and 60's. Therefore what characteristics predisposed children and some adults to these illnesses, given that most individuals exposed to those poisons did not develop symptoms of paralysis and neurological damage? Researchers found a combination of the following factors in cases of what later became classified as paralytic poliomyelitis.

> ➢ High intake of sugar
> ➢ History of long-term antibiotics
> ➢ Recent history of vaccination
> ➢ Tonsillectomy
> ➢ Appendectomy

All of the above factors are in fact immune poisons and/or immune suppressive.

> ➢ Sugar stressing the liver and pancreas. Also affecting the acidity of the blood and other tissues which predisposes mineral loss, tissue breakdown and microbe proliferation. Sugar also affecting brown adipose tissue known to have a role in heat metabolism and therefore fever production. The levels of sugar were extremely high in the summer months when knowledge of the impact of diet was minimal.
> ➢ Antibiotics upset the natural microbial balance of the body promoting the increase in disease causing microbes.
> ➢ Vaccines suppress preliminary defences and are incredibly toxic to the blood and internal tissues.
> ➢ Tonsils and appendix part of the lymphatic system which act to, absorb excess blood toxins, filter and attract white blood cells to destroy and eliminate disease causing agents.

In previous chapters we have discussed the basic function of the immune system in eliminating toxins from the body and maintaining an appropriate microbial system within the external tracts of the body; respiratory, digestive, urinary and external skin. We have also noted the implications of suppressing attempts to eliminate toxins and maintain the membranes with associated microbes, if these functions are extensively compromised as would be the case in individuals with a number of the above predisposing factors then toxins and microbes will eventually invade the internal systems of the body, the most precious and highly guarded system appears to be the nervous system.

The advent of paralytic poliomyelitis coincides with the use of environmental poisons used as insecticides on our food, as with most environmental poisons they would affect the most susceptible first, the most susceptible were found to be the most immune compromised i.e. those with a history of suppression and immune failure; it does in no way correspond to the transfer of virus from one unsuspecting diseased patient to another. The virus has been found to be present in most of us; in fact, as previously discussed, we know that the polio virus belongs to a family of viruses that inhabit the digestive tract, of which we have identified at least 72. Pharmaceutical companies have produced a vaccine supposedly against only 3 of them.

The invasive illnesses as manifest in cases of paralytic poliomyelitis, meningitis, and encephalitis are illnesses where poisons and microbes from the external systems, e.g. the gut, invade the blood and ultimately the brain and nervous system. Viruses themselves as distinct from bacteria can also be created in the internal tissues of the body by the effects of severe poisons such as DDT. If you poison your cells with chemical agents then those very cells will produce viruses.

Paralytic poliomyelitis, acute flaccid paralysis, infantile paralysis, meningitis, encephalitis are illnesses where toxins and microbes penetrate the membranes of the body affecting the internal systems, they are caused in deficient immune systems with an inability to eliminate severe poisons; once this state has been reached then any number of toxins and microbes can penetrate and affect the internal nervous system and brain. Obviously if one is susceptible to these kinds of illnesses it is imperative that you do not expose the body to dangerous toxins, as this would precipitate in an illness that could become invasive, note that it is not possible to avoid exposure to viruses or bacteria as there are billions of these already in the various tracts of the body.

It may be possible to identify different microbes that have been associated with these invasive illnesses, Hib, E.Coli, meningococcal A, B or C, classifying illnesses according to each specific microbe. But conditions with different microbes may be identical to each other and cannot be simply classified according to the name of one particular microbe, viral conditions are different from bacterial and different from fungal, but within those groups the exact nature of the pathology will be a direct function of the host.

Different classes of microbes may create different classes of illness, for example bacterial invasion is usually more severe than viral. The size of the bacterium being much larger than a virus and therefore the bacterial invasion being indicative of a more serious invasive problem than a viral illness, as with viral or bacterial meningitis (inflammation of the membranes around the brain and spinal cord), bacterial is often associated with bacterial septicaemia (proliferation of bacteria in the blood).

It is also important to realise that many other illnesses can lead to invasive complications such as blindness, deafness, paralysis, meningitis, encephalitis and even death. For example any one of the illnesses classified as the developmental illnesses (measles, mumps and chickenpox) and the environmental illnesses (typhoid, cholera and hepatitis) could in fact lead to invasive illnesses with severe consequences. They can all become invasive if not resolved; in fact this is the major concern of all health practitioners when dealing with microbial illnesses. In this way illnesses of the above two categories can change into an illness of the third category, the immune deficient or invasive.

In developing countries the death rate due to measles is much higher than in developed countries, and as reported in Paediatrics (Vol.85 No.2 P.188-94 Feb 1990), studies show a direct link to socio-economic factors. When there are improvements in living conditions, survival rates increase dramatically. Note that in the UK the death rate of measles declined from, approximately **1200** per million **to 6** per million, **before vaccines were introduced** and showed every sign of continuing that declining trend.

As reported in Paediatric Infectious Disease (8:197-200, 1989) there is also orthodox research that shows that vaccines may change the nature of the disease but just as many children go on to die of illnesses with a different classification.

In developing countries when a child is mal -nourished and exposed to severely unhygienic conditions then obviously the amount of toxicity in the child's system is high and the nutritional status is poor, therefore the child's ability to eliminate toxins and microbes that have traversed the membranes of the digestive tract is very much impaired. Therefore unresolved measles illness is more common, they internalise more readily causing neurological complications such as deafness, blindness and meningitis and may even cause death. Vaccines do not of course alleviate this situation but can of course add to the burden which is why immune compromised children are not allowed to be vaccinated.

This is a situation where the trauma is too great and the reactive ability of the patient is too weak, the reason that vaccines don't help, is that they do not aid the immune system to learn, they have wrongly focussed on trying to stimulate an immune memory to viruses and in fact add to the individual's toxicity. The measles virus if isolated and classified would be exactly the same as the measles virus that will be found in a child with few or even imperceptible symptoms in the developed world, the illness is not dangerous by virtue of the microbe but by virtue of the patient.

What is the trauma and what are the susceptibility issues of a child in the developing world? These could be anything from an accumulation of poisons as a result of hygiene issues, exposure to insecticides (that are banned in the developed world), mal-nutrition, vaccines, over-use and inappropriate medication, dehydration, severe emotional trauma, bereavement, physical hardship and so on.

In order to help the child, nutritional deficiencies have to be corrected, for example as reported in the British Medical Journal, (294:294-296, 1987 - Barclay AJ, Foster A, Sommer A. - *Vitamin A supplements and mortality related to measles: a randomized clinical trial)* **vitamin A** supplementation reduces the mortality rate by **seven times** in under 2 year olds, and many studies show increase eye problems and deaths in children with vitamin A deficiency. Rehydration with clean water will be necessary, social and life-style issues have to be addressed and so on. However, to suppress the fever or the skin rash would make the process harder, to vaccinate addresses none of the disease factors hence children go on to die of other illnesses and will be pre-disposed to invasive consequences as a result of the vaccination itself.

The adverse events associated with measles, is not because the measles virus is more "virulent" it is <u>identical</u> to the measles virus that an individual in a developed country eliminates resolving their issues of toxicity leading to immune strengthening. Death rate due to measles **reduce by over 99% before measles vaccine was introduced in UK** because of the factors of diet, sanitation, hygiene, other environmental and living conditions improved, the results of which are unequivocal, both in history and in the present day epidemiology of developing countries.

Therefore how is it possible that apparently healthy children in the developed countries of Europe, USA, Australia, albeit a very small percentage, can also suffer adverse effects from illnesses such as measles?

By referring back to our chronic disease chart it is possible to see how we become susceptible to a range of illnesses according to our history of disease and whether or not these illnesses were resolved, i.e. our history of immune success or failure. As already described, if we experience acute microbial illnesses that are not resolved, then our health level drops into chronic disease patterns, so for example from skin illnesses (as in the psoric miasm) to glandular and lung illnesses (of the tubercular miasm). Vaccines, anti-pyretics, antibiotics, anti-inflammatories, anti-histamines, steroids, broncho-dilators all work against the immune function of the body and can predispose us to immune failure.

The naturopathic tradition of treating measles as documented in "The Hygienic care of children" by Herbert M Shelton and states:

> "...that the invasive consequences and other complications of measles must **all** be the results of <u>suppressive treatment</u>, since they **never** develop under Hygienic (naturopathic) care...This is evidence from an orthodox source, that complications are due to suppressing the eliminative effort through the skin – the rash."

We also know that these patterns are inherited which makes it more imperative that these issues are resolved in the next generation, however with further vaccination and symptom suppression, the subsequent generations will actually start off with even lower levels of health and will not be able to tolerate much more suppression before they become seriously ill. These individuals may not show apparent symptoms of disease, but that is because their symptoms have been suppressed and they are in fact unable to express many symptoms of disease of the higher miasms, many individuals are therefore sensitised to all sorts of poisons and in fact are sensitised to all kinds of foods that now become deadly poisons.

Subsequently, with a minimum of suppression, a potentially mild illness in such individuals of low health will become invasive very quickly, leading to severe neurological complications and even the death of the patient. The orthodox media portray this as the death of an individual that was previously healthy, from a virulent microbe, to which the health profession are racing to create a new vaccine for, with which we will soon be pressured by fear of death to vaccinate with, in order to save the lives of ourselves and our children, when in fact nothing could be further from the truth.

We know that these microbes are present in all of us but only invade the internal systems of individuals that are immune compromised and therefore have unresolved illnesses, and often from previous generations. Vaccines in fact add to the immune burden and predispose us to the very syndromes we are trying to avoid and this becomes more apparent in the immune compromised.

This is why mercury poisoning affects people that have a family history of immune compromised illness, this is also why autism is not spread across the population randomly and evenly, autism occurs in individuals with a family history of immune compromised illness, autism often affects more than one child in the same family. This is also why illnesses of the carcinosin miasm, for example cancer, occurs now at younger ages than ever before in children with a history of cancer in previous generations, these are all indicative of unresolved patterns of illness that are passed on to subsequent generations.

Illnesses are multifactorial, there are many factors and they affect individuals according to their susceptibility, for example many of us are aware of the dangers of smoking but smoking does not cause lung cancer with the first cigarette, some may never develop cancer, but smoking, although may have short-term benefits for some will also have longer term disadvantages that only become apparent in time and appear more frequently in the most susceptible.

How can we be so sure? Well the proof of the pudding comes from the observation of patients. Here we see that a curative reaction, wherein symptoms move;

> *from either up to down, inside to out, from more important organs to less important organs, in reverse order of appearance, liberating increasing physical, mental and emotional energy,*

…occurs when the healing response is helped not suppressed. For individuals with chronic disease, after successful treatment, we see the phenomenon of the 'return of old symptoms', symptoms of illness that were not resolved reappearing briefly resulting in a curative response. Once we have a map of illness we can see how far the patient is deteriorating or improving, we are able to see what factors aid health and what adds to the deterioration of health.

For example:

If after a vaccine a child develops eczema, the use of steroid cream could suppress the inflammatory condition and leave the child with asthma, further use of inhaled steroids and bronchodilators could eventually lead to allergic reactions and after a period of stress and anxiety an episode of glandular fever and if not resolved could lead to chronic fatigue with leaky membranes, immunoglobulin nephropathy etc. Each subsequent condition is a deterioration of the previous and of course in no way is the patient able to do anything as eliminative as measles. After holistic treatment, for example using homeopathy, we would expect to see from the chronic glandular fever acute inflammatory reaction and the return of a chest condition, treating acute chest reactions successfully would bring back the symptoms of eczema, the successful treatment of which would leave the patient susceptible to acute eliminative rashes and with no allergic sensitivities to environmental proteins and foods.

Once we know our medical history, that of our parents and grandparents, we can predict to some degree the kind of illnesses we are susceptible to. Serious illness does not happen for 'no reason' in perfectly healthy people and is not the responsibility of the microbe. The only way a healthy person can get a serious illness is from a serious and most obvious trauma; a serious trauma being a large dose of poison, exposure to high dose radiation, difficult bereavement, extended period of mal-nutrition, severe physical injury. A serious trauma is not a serious microbe, microbes are neither serious nor not serious, bacteria in your colon, is a sign of health but the same bacteria in your blood is a sign of a serious problem.

If we therefore look at polio and illustrate what happens in different individuals, we can see that the pattern of illness is very dependent on the susceptibility of the individual. Looking at our health level chart, those at the top will display no symptoms at all even though they are exposed to the same poison and nucleic acids believed to be from polio can be detected in the digestive tract. Further down the levels, individuals with the same exposure to poison will show symptoms perhaps of vomiting and diarrhoea, further down in health there may be a generalised inflammatory response, further down some mild invasive symptoms with paralysis lasting for no more than 24 hours, down again and we see individuals with symptoms of paralysis lasting for longer, perhaps with muscle wasting that is recoverable, down further still symptoms of long term paralysis and down to the lowest levels of health and we see brain damage and even death.

All illnesses, all scenarios are possible, the difference between individuals may be due to two things, one being the level of trauma and the second their level of health. The viral DNA is in fact a constant in all cases; it is not primarily responsible for the disease or the severity of the disease. You may ask; surely some viruses and bacteria are so dangerous that very few people survive their illnesses regardless of how healthy you are?

15.3 What about dangerous viruses?

15.3.1 Spanish Flu

Much of the impetus to the current measures to combat current illnesses for example, Bird Flu, Sars and Swine Flu etc comes from scientists' fear of a recurrence of an epidemic similar to the 1918 Spanish Flu. An epidemic is an illness prevalent at one particular time affecting a national area. A pandemic affects large populations of the world at one time and the 1918 flu was a severe pandemic with a large death toll said to be due to a flu virus rampaging throughout much of Europe and eventually across the rest of the world.

In reality there were numerous reasons why the flu of the 1918 winter would have been more severe than any other. Firstly we were at the end of the First World War with a massive death toll, family bereavement and separation, appalling living conditions, malnutrition and unprecedented levels of fear.

Patients suffered from dehydration which would have been enough to kill them during any illness with a fever. Doctors were brought out of retirement to cope with illnesses because so many younger doctors were involved in the war, these replacement doctors would have been trained in the 1880's and were using very old and ineffective treatment methods. Reports show many patients had symptoms of aspirin overdose and side-effects from experimental vaccines and anti-sera.

In addition people were displaying many different kinds of symptoms and these illnesses were given various disease names, eventually they lumped all of those illnesses together as Spanish Flu, but the symptoms were in no way consistent. It is only in retrospect that researchers are guesstimating that this could have been a viral illness but we have to remember that in 1918 we had no way of isolating and classifying viruses.

Recent attempts to classify the 1918 flu virus have come from isolating pieces of genetic information (not actually isolating the virus) from a body that was approximately 90 years old; a diseased body that would have been filled with all kinds of dead cells, contaminant, microbes and genetic information. Then with the aid of laboratory techniques and computer simulation some scientists have tried to predict what the viral DNA and virus would have been like and subsequently guess what microscopic virus was responsible for millions of deaths in 1918.

The 1918 Spanish Flu that some vaccine promoters are saying could return if a virulent virus attacked, could only happen if the world's population descended into a situation similar to the living conditions prevalent in 1918. The death toll was entirely related to the susceptibility of the individuals living at the end of the First World War and not due to a particularly strong flu virus that wanted to kill as many people as possible. The fear of a repeat of the 1918 flu pandemic is borne out of a medical perception that views disease as something that has nothing to do with the patient, their susceptibility or their living conditions.

Neither was the high death toll due to a novel virus that we had no prior immunity to. A pandemic of the proportions of the 1918 incidentally, has never materialised again, in spite of the frequency of viral mutations and likelihood of creating new viruses that we have no immunity to and despite dire warnings from the pharmaceutical industry encouraging wave upon wave of successive vaccination programs.

15.3.2 Ebola

Ebola received a lot of publicity in its early days, a devastating disease resulting in external and internal bleeding often leading to death. An illness of which we have no treatment, no knowledge of where the virus normally inhabits, but often associated with health-care facilities and one form can also occur in monkeys, gorillas and chimpanzees. This Ebola-Reston virus was supposed to cause severe illness and death in monkeys imported to research facilities in the United States and Italy from the Philippines; during these outbreaks, several research workers became infected with the virus, but did not become ill.

An illness so devastating, caused by a virus capable of killing anyone in its path, at least that's what the public have been led to believe and yet we have no treatment or vaccine, which raises the question, why hasn't it killed everyone in its path? The source of the virus is unknown; therefore quarantine would only be possible once the patient had symptoms, why is the disease not spreading from whence it came? A quote from the Centre for Disease Control (special pathogens branch) sheds a different light: - "researchers do not understand why some people are able to recover and some do not". Clearly this is also a case of individual susceptibility, without further research there is much about the illness that remains unknown, however it is interesting to know that it usually spreads within healthcare facilities which are of course immune suppression facilities and in laboratory animals as opposed to other animals in captivity.

15.3.3 Bird Flu

And so to Bird Flu, reminding me of the saying 'if you want to know the truth, follow the money'…The story is the same, individuals becoming ill and dying, we find evidence of a possible virus in their system and we say that is the cause of their death. The problem is however, how do we know that the virus is not an effect rather than the cause? Viruses are species specific, meaning that humans do not replicate bird viruses; the illness has only appeared in those in close contact with birds, bird viruses found in humans may have been found as a result of contamination but have no role in pathology. The living conditions of livestock are important factors in their disease and therefore in the formation of viruses, more important than the theory of catching a disease from the transmission of a virus from another bird, why are we not looking at those conditions when assessing the factors responsible for disease? Why should we be more concerned of the bird flu virus mutating to a human form as compared to any other animal virus on the planet? Birds in captivity are also subject to poisoning which could create viruses; they are also subject to vaccination which does create mutant viruses. Laboratories are in fact altering these bird flu viruses (for example AH5N1) with human influenza viruses, what are the possible implications with regard to vaccinations in humans and live-stock?

Patricia A. Doyle, DVM, PhD., Tropical Agricultural Economics.

> *"I have been plotting outbreaks for almost two years, using migration maps and studying bird flyways, etc. Well, I noticed something different this season. The winter bird migrations did NOT bring bird flu with the migratory birds. Cases should NOW be breaking out in Africa, Malawi and other countries that host winter migratory birds. Well, the bird flu does not seem to be where it is supposed to be i.e. going by the past migrations…are the re-emerging outbreaks in china, Vietnam, Russia, Romania etc. occurring due to vaccinations?"*

We have already mentioned Dr Marc Girard's condemnation of the WHO promotion of a flu vaccine against a predicted pandemic of bird flu:

> *"As a result, experts are currently challenging the WHO on the fact that deporting a veterinarian issue to a medical one prevented national agencies from taking appropriate measures concerning animals which, most probably, would have been far more efficient in limiting the spread of epidemics. In addition, it is sufficient to consider the figures of fatal reports following flu vaccination (Scrip n° 3101, p. 6) and to have a minimum of familiarity with the problem of under-reporting, to understand that up till now* **irresponsible vaccination against flu has killed far more people than avian (bird) flu."**

And to follow the money, Donald Rumsfeld, USA Secretary of State holds shares in the company 'Gilead' that owns the rights to the so-called anti-viral drug 'Tamiflu', which is being produced under license by the Swiss Pharmaceutical 'Roche', promoted as the drug of choice in any forth coming bird flu epidemic. October 2005, Nelson D. Schwartz, senior writer of the USA business magazine 'Fortune' reports:

> "Rumsfeld served as Gilead Research's chairman from 1997 until he joined the Bush administration in 2001 and he still holds a Gilead stake valued at between $5 million and $25 million, according to federal financial disclosures filed by Rumsfeld. The forms don't reveal the exact number of shares Rumsfeld owns, but in the past six months fears of a pandemic and the ensuing scramble for Tamiflu have sent Gilead's stock from $35 to $47. That's made the Pentagon chief, already one of the wealthiest members of the Bush cabinet, ***at least $1 million richer.***"

Did the pandemic materialise, millions of cases, 1,000's dead? No, it did not, we are of course still waiting for the pandemic, 6 months later however, what did materialise for Donald Rumsfeld?

March 2006, Geoffrey Lean and Jonathan Owen report in the UK newspaper 'The Independent'.

> *"Donald Rumsfeld has made a killing out of bird flu. The US Defence Secretary has made more than $5m (£2.9m) in capital gains from selling shares in the biotechnology firm that discovered and developed Tamiflu, the drug being bought in massive amounts by Governments to treat a possible human pandemic of the disease."*

So, is the bird flu panic lead by scientific evidence? Apparently not, at least according to a report in the British Medical Journal, Oct 2005, (331: 975 – 976).

> *"The lack of sustained human-to-human transmission suggests that this AH5N1 avian virus (the bird flu virus) does not currently have the capacity to cause a human pandemic"*

15.3.4 HIV

What about illnesses such as HIV you may say, surely we have a formidable and virulent pathogen indiscriminately attacking and killing those that it happens to infect. From the old infectious disease perspective this may appear to be the case and is certainly promoted as such by the popular press and the proponents of mainstream pharmaceutical approaches to disease management. An analysis of the research is in fact very straight forward in those with a minimum of research background, but a very large subject and too large to do justice to in this book, however I shall quote from the numerous and eminent scientists that are fully aware that the disease phenomena, Acquired Immune Deficiency Syndrome (AIDS), cannot be attributable to a single virus, HIV or any other.

Many scientists within the field of virology and AIDS research have always questioned the role of the newly discovered retrovirus HIV as the causation of the illness AIDS. Indeed after several years of research many are convinced that HIV is not in fact the cause of AIDS and a number of scientists have formed; 'The Group for the Scientific Reappraisal of the HIV-AIDS Hypothesis' and have documented statements and links to research and correspondence stating just that.

Dr. Kary Mullis, Biochemist, 1993 Nobel Prize for Chemistry:

> *"If there is evidence that HIV causes AIDS, there should be scientific documents which either singly or collectively demonstrate that fact, at least with a high probability. There is no such document." (Sunday Times - London, 28 Nov. 1993)*

Dr. Heinz Ludwig Sänger, Emeritus Professor of Molecular Biology and Virology, Max-Planck-Institutes for Biochemistry, München. Robert Koch Award 1978:

> *"Up to today there is actually no single scientifically really convincing evidence for the existence of HIV. Not even once such a retrovirus has been isolated and purified by the methods of classical virology." (Letter to Süddeutsche Zeitung 2000)*

Dr. Serge Lang, Professor of Mathematics, Yale University:

> *"I do not regard the causal relationship between HIV and any disease as settled. I have seen considerable evidence that highly improper statistics concerning HIV and AIDS have been passed off as science, and that top members of the scientific establishment have carelessly, if not irresponsibly, joined the media in spreading misinformation about the nature of AIDS." (Yale Scientific, Fall 1994)*

Dr. Harvey Bialy, Molecular Biologist, former editor of *Bio/Technology* and *Nature Biotechnology*:

> *"HIV is an ordinary retrovirus. There is nothing about this virus that is unique. Everything that is discovered about HIV has an*

analogue in other retroviruses that don't cause AIDS. HIV only contains a very small piece of genetic information. There's no way it can do all these elaborate things they say it does." (Spin June 1992)

Dr. Gordon Stewart, Emeritus Professor of Public Health, University of Glasgow:

"AIDS is a behavioural disease. It is multifactorial, brought on by several simultaneous strains on the immune system - drugs, pharmaceutical and recreational, sexually transmitted diseases, multiple viral infections." (Spin June 1992)

Dr. Charles Thomas, former Professor of Biochemistry, Harvard and John Hopkins Universities:

"The HIV-causes-AIDS dogma represents the grandest and perhaps the most morally destructive fraud that has ever been perpetrated on young men and women of the Western world." (Sunday Times (London) 3 April 1994)

Dr. Joseph Sonnabend, New York Physician, founder of the American Foundation for AIDS Research (AmFAR):

"The marketing of HIV, through press releases and statements, as a killer virus causing AIDS without the need for any other factors, has so distorted research and treatment that it may have caused thousands of people to suffer and die." (Sunday times (London) 17 May 1992)

Dr. Etienne de Harven, Emeritus Professor of Pathology, at the University of Toronto:

"Dominated by the media, by special pressure groups and by the interests of several pharmaceutical companies, the AIDS establishment efforts to control the disease lost contact with open-minded, peer-reviewed medical science since the

*unproven HIV/AIDS hypothesis received 100% of the research
funds while all other hypotheses were ignored." (Reappraising
AIDS Nov. /Dec. 1998)*

Dr. Bernard Forscher, former editor of the U.S. *Proceeding of the
National Academy of Sciences*:

> *"The HIV hypothesis ranks with the 'bad air' theory for malaria
> and the 'bacterial infection' theory of beriberi and pellagra
> [caused by nutritional deficiencies]. It is a hoax that became a
> scam." (Sunday Times (London) 3 April 1994)*

Not only are there problems with the HIV causes AIDS hypothesis but
astoundingly the evidence for the existence of the newly discovered
retrovirus HIV is almost entirely non-existent. Researchers have been
working with what they think the retrovirus is doing (i.e. reverse
transcription) without ever having isolated and therefore found the virus.
In addition when diagnosing someone with having the virus HIV
positive, they are in fact detecting antibodies to a protein that they
believe is from the virus.

Electron microscopy of the relevant portions of the cells that contain the
virus is a minimal requirement of identification; Dr Etienne de Harven is
emeritus Professor of Pathology, University of Toronto. He worked in
electron microscopy (EM) primarily on the ultra-structure of retroviruses
throughout his professional career of 25 years at the Sloan Kettering
Institute in New York and 13 years at the University of Toronto.
Regarding HIV research and the lack of electron microscopy studies he
has this to say:

> *"It is only in 1997, after fifteen years of intensive HIV research,
> that elementary EM (electron microscopy) controls were
> performed, with the disastrous results recently reviewed in
> Continuum. How many wasted efforts, how many billions of
> research dollars gone in smoke ...**Horrible.**"*

The disastrous results were the first electron micrographs i.e. highly magnified pictures of portions of cell extracts supposed to be containing isolated virus and the discovery that most of the contents was in fact cell debris and smaller particles without the structure of retroviruses. This is what researchers were using as isolated HIV retrovirus.

Most of the scientific community accept what they are being told by other researchers; most of the non-research scientific community including health professionals accept likewise, and therefore the public, way down the information line, accept what is being perpetuated by the media, hook, line and sinker. When researchers do their own investigating they are often surprised:

Dr. Heinz Ludwig Sänger, Emeritus Professor of Molecular Biology and Virology and a former director of the Department of Viroid Research at the Max-Planck-Institutes for Biochemy near München,

> *"During the past 20 years HIV-AIDS research has shown to a line of critical scientists again and again that the existence of HIV has not been proven without doubt and that both from an aetiological (causal), and an epidemiological view, it cannot be responsible for the immunodeficiency AIDS. In view of the general accepted HIV/AIDS hypothesis **this appeared to me so unbelievable that I decided to investigate it myself.** After three years of intensive and, above all, critical studies of the relevant original literature, as an experienced virologist and molecular biologist I came to the following surprising conclusion: **Up to today there is actually no single scientifically really convincing evidence for the existence of HIV.** Not even once such a retrovirus has been isolated and purified by the methods of classical virology."*

We are of course no different, what choice do we have other than to believe what the scientific community appear to be telling us, albeit through the mechanism of the media. It is therefore important to realise that the HIV/AIDS theory, the theory that you can catch AIDS by catching the HIV retrovirus, is just a theory, to which many scientists do not adhere to and of which the evidence for is entirely lacking. However, the counter story, even though scientifically more dominant, does not get media attention

Time again throughout history we have witnessed the advent of a disease that is promoted as being caused by a powerful disease agent, something that exists outside of us, that has nothing to do with our own susceptibility, when in fact research shows quite the opposite. In spite of this, research finances are poured into attempting to find the 'one' external microbial cause, so that we can profitably produce the magic bullet and administer cure without the need to take responsibility for a single contributing disease factor. Meanwhile the real factors that determine health and disease are side-lined; toxicity, nutritional deficiency, suppressed elimination, immune suppression, emotional abuse, emotional suppression and drug use.

AIDS is not in fact a single disease, there are many different symptoms and it is classified differently in different countries, there are now syndromes that look like AIDS that are now called ARC (AIDS related complex). The attachment to a belief that disease is caused by an external germ is so strong that it can defy rationality.

> *"The 'rules' employed by HIV/AIDS researchers, that is, detection of a protein, p24, OR an enzyme, reverse transcriptase, do not satisfy any scientific principle proving isolation of a viral particle and indeed **defy common sense"**.*

Written by Dr Eleni Papadopulos-Eleopulos, Professor of medical physics and Dr David Causer, Senior physicist, head of medical physics, both at Royal Perth Hospital together with Dr Valendar Turner, Professor of emergency medicine and Dr John Papadimitriou, Practicing pathologist and Professor at University both of Western Australia's medical school, in response to the claim that HIV has been found in AIDS patients.

Research shows AIDS is not sexually transmitted

In 1997 Nancy Padian published research in The American Journal of Epidemiology the results of which were even more incongruent with the HIV AIDS theory. From 1985 to 1995 a total of 82 infected women and their male partners and 360 infected men and their female partners (all non-injection drug users) were recruited from health care providers, research studies, and health departments throughout Northern California, and they were interviewed and examined at various study clinic sites.

> *"To our knowledge, our study is the largest and longest study of the heterosexual transmission of HIV in the United States. The consistency of results over the 10-year duration argues for the validity of our results."*

N.Padian Am J Epidemiol Vol. 146, No. 4, 1997

The results showed that over the 10 year study period **NOBODY** became HIV positive from their partners, despite having long-term and often non-protective sexual relationships.

> *Nevertheless, the absence of seroincident infection over the course of the study cannot be entirely attributed to significant behaviour change. No transmission occurred among the 25 percent of couples who did not use condoms consistently at their last follow-up nor among the 47 couples who intermittently practiced unsafe sex during the entire duration of follow-up.*

N.Padian Am J Epidemiol Vol. 146, No. 4, 1997

The story of AIDS is an account of disease that once more highlights the ability of those in power to grasp at opportunities to promote their own social agenda and their own financial gain. Similarly, an opportunity for others in research, supported by the same financial institutions, to base investigations that express a limited mind-set, whilst satisfying those that are psychologically attached to a simplistic view of disease, a view that has been promoted since the days of Pasteur.

CHAPTER 15 - SUMMARY

> ➤ Infectious disease manifests according to a patients susceptibility of which the microbe plays a secondary role.

> ➤ The immune system is not just an attack and defend system, but is involved in eliminating toxins and balancing the eco-system of microbial cells and our own cells

> ➤ Immune development is not just about the ability to recognise our cells and foreign cells but involves our ability to deal with the environment and is intimately connected to all physical, mental and emotional development.

> ➤ Infectious diseases can be classified according to the nature of the patient as well as the associated microbe; developmental, environmental and immune compromised.

> ➤ With our broader understanding of disease we realise that the two boys of the famous smallpox experiments of Edward Jenner; James Phipps and Edward Jenner's son, both died of tuberculosis which was predisposed by the vaccine. They did not develop the rash of smallpox, but due to the nature of the blood poisoning induced by the vaccination, their disease was in fact driven deeper, and far from being immunised they were in fact immune compromised.

> ➤ Microbes themselves are neither safe nor dangerous and they are only associated with illnesses that relate to the susceptibility of the patient.

CHAPTER SIXTEEN

16 What exactly do vaccines do?

The vaccine issue is often a highly emotive one and there are many scare tactics used to promote vaccines, as with many commercial products. People often have numerous questions and unresolved issues about vaccines, not least because there is also a large body of non-expert 'experts' in the shape of family, friends and the media, offering their admonishments and advice.

It is a topic that needs a little investigation but I believe the subject of this book provides a very sound basis for understanding the underlying principles, and therefore hopefully making it much easier to come to a reasoned and confident conclusion.

I shall provide a summary of some of the main issues relating to how vaccines affect the body. However, once the main issues are understood, many people still have questions that ultimately relate to how and why so much of the established medical community remain invested in vaccines, i.e. what of the laboratory tests, trials, evidence, statistics, epidemiology, safety studies, etc.

This has been a special interest of mine for many years starting with the original publication of my booklet 'Mass Immunisation: A point in question' written in 1989, but for additional detail please refer to the more recent book 'VACCINES – This book could remove the fear of childhood illnesses' - Trevor Gunn, where I do go into all of those issues in more depth.

By looking at the bigger picture as well as the detail it is possible to see how vaccines suppress and sensitise the immune system to the contents of the vaccine. They therefore can create more problems than they solve and consequently appear to work by sometimes reducing one type of sickness but increase your susceptibility to other illnesses.

16.1 The inherent risks of vaccination

The strategies of the priesthood in defending the human from attacking entities, create castles, weapons and creeds of conduct to protect us, but of course restrict and eventually kill us, imposing its belief system on the enemy it becomes the enemy, it even affects those that resist, for resistance is part of the problem.

The vaccine elements are injected into the body, past the body's normal lines of defence, (exceptions being the oral vaccines, polio being the most common, although the UK schedule has recently changed to an injectable form). There are many ways of injecting; intravenously, subcutaneously, intramuscularly etc, vaccines are not injected intravenously and so some medical professionals believe that vaccines are therefore not injected into the blood. However, all injections including the intramuscular and subcutaneous will give access of their contents directly to the blood system as the skin, in all instances of injection, will be pierced and therefore the immune functions of the skin are bypassed.

16.2 Vaccines bypass most of the immune system

Vaccine producers claim to be stimulating the immune system when clearly they are not; most of the immune system is by-passed, vaccine producers are pre-occupied with stimulating a blood antibody response to viruses, microbes and toxins which is in fact highly illogical given the following:

> We **do not know** how or whether a virus causes an illness, viral causation is still a theory, and yet we do know that poisoning a cell creates viruses, therefore vaccine promoters cannot say that they have found the cause of a disease when they find indirect evidence of genetic material thought to be from a virus.

> We **do not know** the best immune response to these pathogens, therefore why are vaccine producers so concerned with creating blood anti-bodies, when other systems may be far more important?

> We **do know** that in individuals with poor immune function; - AIDS, allergies, asthma and autoimmune disease - their immune response favours anti-body production instead of the cellular response. Therefore why are we trying to create anti-bodies and effectively mimic the situation of immune dysfunction?

> We **do know** that children incapable of producing antibodies overcome illnesses and obtain immunity far better than children with poor cellular immunity, if antibodies do not appear to be as important as the cellular response, why are we not concerned with stimulating cellular immunity but instead pre-occupied with creating anti-bodies?

The practice of vaccination for the purpose of creating blood anti-bodies is in fact highly questionable. However, if in fact vaccine promoters acknowledge that whatever the mechanism is for immunity, the hope is that the vaccine will stimulate a similar enough response to allow immune learning and a reduced susceptibility to future illness. Then the second point to consider is how similar to an illness is the response to vaccination?

Having injected the vaccine components into the blood, the stimulation of a blood immune response (generally considered to be the creation of antibodies) is often thought of as being sufficient to create immunity.

However, regardless of what immune elements are stimulated in the blood, a **successful** immune response does **not** just require the formation of antibodies or any other immune cells within the blood system; a successful immune response necessarily involves the successful **elimination** of the toxins and microbes. Any health professional that thinks the mere production of antibodies is indicative of an effective immune response does not understand immune 'processes'.

> *Mario Clerci of the National Cancer Institute in the US suggests: ...that by looking at HIV positive patients i.e. the ones that are producing antibodies, we're looking at the immune failures.*

In fact most individuals that are vaccinated do not seem to respond at all with visible symptoms, for some this may be indicative of sufficient health and minimal sensitivity to the components of the vaccines, for others this could be indicative of an inability to eliminate toxins and therefore an increased immune load and greater susceptibility to future illness.

Essentially it is hoped that the vaccine will cause the body to create antibodies, even though, immunologists have to admit to not knowing the precise mechanism of the immune response to viruses, or for that matter any other pathogen.

The hope is of course that whatever the mechanism is, the action of the vaccine will stimulate a similar enough response in order to prime the body for any subsequent attack. But here we immediately run into significant problems, the injection of many vaccine pathogens alone actually stimulates little or no apparent immune response in the blood – antibodies or otherwise.

16.3 A spoon full of poison – helps the medicine go down

In fact, in order for some vaccines to stimulate the immune system to any significant degree a substance called an **adjuvant** is added to the vaccine contents. An adjuvant is a chemical that will stimulate an immune response; it is therefore toxic to the human body and is effectively a **poison**. Without this poison the vaccine doesn't have a significantly measurable antibody response. The most common adjuvant is aluminium, a heavy metal with known toxic effects on the nervous system.

Why does the body <u>not</u> mount a significant immune response to the elements of the vaccine?

It does sound rather strange, that if we have made for example a diphtheria, tetanus, Hib meningitis, hepatitis B, DPT, Pediacel 5 in 1 vaccine, why does the body not produce a significant immune response to the elements of the vaccine without having to add another poison? There may be several reasons for this:

> Here we may come to the understanding that actually the live, attenuated or killed pathogen does not pose a significant or <u>apparent</u> threat to the human body; by the reactions, or rather lack of reaction, of the human body to these vaccine pathogens, it would appear that they may not be the real cause of illnesses.
> The lack of reaction to the vaccine pathogens may be as a result of changing the pathogen in the process of making the vaccine; it is possible that the vaccine components do not significantly mirror the real virus, microbe or toxin.
> In addition, illnesses in their natural form would arise from a natural build-up of toxins and microbes on the outer membranes of your body or from an obvious injury. You would be alerted to a problem and would already be mounting an inflammatory response; infiltration of these elements into the blood will be quickly followed by a blood immune response that

will make every attempt to eliminate these toxic elements. However a vaccine bypasses most of this response and may have tricked your body into accepting toxins without a response.

> But it may also be possible that the body is reacting to the contents of the vaccine, with other immune cells and NOT antibodies. BUT because only antibodies are measured when testing the effects of the vaccine. Vaccines are only considered to be effective if measurable amounts of antibodies are detected. Therefore dangerous chemical agents are placed in vaccines to **_force_** the body to produce antibodies.

Unfortunately proper controlled studies that test for the safety and effectiveness of vaccines are not conducted, although they are of course carried out for nearly all other pharmaceutical products.

The Cochrane Collaboration was set up in 1992 by the UK National Health Service Research and Development Program to assess trials published in peer reviewed scientific journals, the head of the Vaccines Division is Tom Jefferson, writing in the British Medical Journal he states:

> "The inception of a vaccination campaign seems to preclude the assessment of a vaccine through placebo controlled randomised trials on ethical grounds. Far from being unethical, however, such trials are desperately needed and we should invest in them without delay. A further consequence is reliance on non-randomised studies once the campaign is under way. It is debatable whether these can contribute to our understanding of the effectiveness of vaccines."
>
> BMJ (333: 912-915) 28 Oct 2006

16.4 How vaccines start a chain reaction of symptoms, drug escalation and serious illness.

"If the only tool you have is a hammer, you tend to see every problem as a nail."

Abraham Maslow

By vaccinating we are in fact injecting a potentially dangerous cocktail of poisons and possible pathogens into the body, and from what we know of our immune system, we would therefore expect an immune reaction; a reaction designed to minimise the progress of these elements further into the body, eliminate these elements entirely from the body, and ideally have learnt from the whole process such that we are now less susceptible to such a natural illness in the future.

The fact is, some individuals do respond with such immune reactions with symptoms of fever, possibly eliminative rashes and mucus production; however, these individuals are then strongly advised, by the same medical advisors administering the vaccines, to **suppress these immune reactions**. Suppress, using pharmaceutical medication such as Calpol etc.

So, having injected dangerous poisons into the body, in order to stimulate an immune response, any reactions designed to resolve the trauma (other than the internal production of antibodies) are then suppressed.

Vaccine promoters must therefore be saying that the blood immune response to vaccine poisons i.e. the production of antibodies, is ok, but any other associated response is not ok and should therefore be suppressed with medication. This is obviously an illogical and in fact very dangerous policy; especially in view of the fact that we **know** how vitally important reactions such as the generalised inflammatory response is, with subsequent rash and toxin elimination, and we don't know how exactly the immune system mounts an effective response to, for example, viruses. Therefore how can one rationalise suppressing aspects of our response, especially those aspects that we **know** are vitally important.

This point cannot be overstated; the whole purpose of vaccination is to stimulate the immune system, yet this is exactly what is being <u>*suppressed*</u> *by the routine use of antipyretic and anti-inflammatory medication such as Calpol or paracetamol after vaccination.*

16.5 The problems persist

By the process of vaccination we are aware that vaccine elements are injected into the blood, which therefore bypasses most of the immune system; often there are no apparent attempts to eliminate these toxins. The body has been effectively tricked into accepting a vast array of toxins that ordinarily it does its utmost to keep out and if there are any reactions, then these are routinely suppressed with medication.

If these vaccine elements remain within the system, then not only do we have the problem of the effect of those poisons and immune complexes in the internal system, but we also have the problems inherent in the issue of **'unresolved'** elimination. We know that <u>unresolved</u> reactions lead to persistent similar reactions, that is to say,

…**Acute reactions that are unsuccessful give rise to persistent chronic reactions.**

What are the possible implications of this with regard to vaccines?

The natural reaction to poisons taken into the blood would be a generalised inflammatory reaction involving dilation (widening) of blood vessels - bringing blood including the white blood cells to the affected area; plus increased permeability (leakiness) of the blood vessel wall and external membranes —allowing waste materials and white blood cells out.

As discussed earlier, this is a purposeful, sophisticated and coordinated response designed to enhance white blood cell destruction of toxins and microbes, with the elimination of waste matter across the membranes of the body. An injection of toxins into the blood from a vaccine that could **not** be eliminated via an acute elimination reaction (i.e. an elimination that would happen in a natural acute disease such as measles) could therefore lead to persistent chronic reactions.

Therefore could vaccination give rise to persistent low-level immune reaction including membrane leaking?

This has in fact been demonstrated and reported by Henry Pabst in the case of MMR vaccination and reported in Vaccine Vol. 15, issue 1, pages 10-14, titled "Kinetics of immunological responses after primary MMR vaccine" demonstrating the persistent presence of immune chemicals such as interferon gamma which has been demonstrated to cause an increased permeability of the membranes of the digestive tract and blood brain barrier. Thus the biological effects of vaccination on the membranes of those vaccinated have been demonstrated, illustrating the nature of the **unresolved** immune reaction that can happen as a consequence of vaccination. In such cases there has been no immune learning, but in fact immune failure.

From what we have discussed of the principles of "learning", an effective immune response, especially those that have been classified as the childhood illnesses, when **resolved,** gives rise to the successful elimination of toxins and microbes and a decreased susceptibility to ingested toxins. The systems become stronger, the membrane becomes **stronger,** (not weaker, i.e. not persistently more permeable as has been demonstrated with vaccines), after the resolution of natural illness we are less susceptible to allowing in other toxins and microbes from our food and environment.

Therefore the blood elimination reaction need only occur enough times to sufficiently strengthen the membranes and associated systems. Consequently we do not need to subject our **blood** to all possible environmental toxins in order to develop antibodies to each and every one of them, what vaccine producers consider to be; 'immunity'.

Vaccinators do not understand the nature of immune learning, like any learning process, you do not need to be subjected to every possible problem to learn how to resolve them. When learning to ride a bike it is not necessary to bruise every surface of the skin or break every possible limb in the learning process. Similarly once you've mastered a right turn, then that's it, you are not going to fall over at every other different right turn you encounter. Similarly once you've learnt a specific toxin and microbe elimination, the nature of immune learning is such that the membrane has the ability to keep out all kinds of other toxins more efficiently than before the learning process.

Individuals with high levels of health that exist from year to year **without** symptoms of colds and flu **do not** have antibodies to all the different viruses and bacteria that are supposedly implicated in these diseases. Their external immune defences function sufficiently well to keep the necessary elements out of their blood system. That is the goal of a fully functional and developed immune system. Note, therefore, with vaccines the opposite has been demonstrated, vaccination injects toxins that are not eliminated from the blood system, creating membranes that are persistently leaky which would therefore lead to **increased susceptibility** to blood toxicity, and an increase in chronic immune reactions.

Far from becoming immune to the vaccine elements, in such instances individuals become **sensitised** to these elements with the added pathology of poor membrane function. Not only do they respond persistently to an ongoing problem but also the nature of the leaky membrane is such that they now allow in a wider range of foods, toxins and microbes. They become more susceptible to such pathogens entering their blood and from the vaccinators frame of reference they have every reason to develop even more vaccines in an attempt to address susceptibility to an infinite possibility of microbes and toxins. This is good news from a commercial point of view for those in the vaccine industry, but bad news for your immune system.

Is there any evidence of this when comparing actual disease rates in vaccinated and non-vaccinated individuals? A report in the Lancet, 29 June 1996 illustrated that studies show children with a history of natural illnesses such as measles, mumps and rubella were less likely to suffer with **allergies** in later life. Researchers from Southampton General Hospital in the UK now confirm this, discovering that:

> *Children with a history of measles suffer less from allergic conditions such as asthma, eczema and hay fever when compared to vaccinated individuals.*

Similarly research by Michel Odent reported in the Journal of the American Medical Association (1994; 272:592-3) showed that the use of whooping cough vaccine increased the incidence of asthma by 5-6 times as compared to non-vaccinated children. This was later confirmed by research at Churchill Hospital in Oxford UK and presented to the British Thoracic Society by Chest Consultant, Dr Julian Hopkin.

If toxins have crossed the membranes of the body and have failed to be eliminated then the individual becomes sensitised to those substances and then has to develop new strategies to prevent any more of those substances entering the body and causing further problems.

16.6 Allergies

Allergies are often thought of as an 'over-sensitivity' to potentially harmless substances. From an orthodox perspective therefore, another example of how the reactions of the body are perceived as 'malfunctions'. When presenting with such a condition we are told that we have an 'over-reactive' immune system, responding to harmless elements that we need not react to, therefore a condition that we need medication to suppress. (See Chapter 9)

16.6.1 Vaccines and allergies

We can demonstrate the potential risks of vaccines because they bypass most of the immune system, leaving the body with the very difficult task of eliminating such poisons. This can therefore lead to <u>unresolved</u> blood toxicity, which in turn leads to, membrane weakness, sensitivities and therefore persistent immune reactions (allergic reactions, such as eczema, asthma and hayfever). We can therefore understand how successful immune reactions such as natural measles, rubella, chicken pox, etc would successfully eliminate toxins leading to membrane strength and a reduced sensitivity to potential allergens.

Consequently we are able to understand the previously quoted study, reported in the Lancet 29 June 1996, showing that children with a history of natural illnesses such as measles, mumps and rubella were less likely to suffer with **allergies** in later life. Researchers from Southampton General Hospital in the UK confirm this, discovering that:

> *Children with a history of measles suffer less from allergic conditions such as asthma, eczema and hay fever when compared to vaccinated individuals.*

By the process of vaccination; we are injecting poisons into the blood of someone that may be unable to eliminate them, this is especially likely in the underdeveloped immune system of a young child, and these specific vaccine components would then provide the source of specific allergies later on. The conclusion of a study into the specific antibody responses to pertussis (whooping cough) vaccine was reported in the European Journal of Paediatrics in 1999:

> *Conclusion: Acellular pertussis immunization induces IgE antibodies to pertussis toxin, especially after booster vaccination.*

Eur J Pediatr. 1999 Dec;158(12):989-94

Thus demonstrating that the IgE antibody reaction, (associated with allergic responses) was as a direct response to the vaccine. With the following components contained in various vaccines; egg, yeast, antibiotics, lactose, gelatine, monosodium glutamate, this does suggest a very plausible mechanism for creating these specific allergies in susceptible people. It is also interesting to note the prevalence of latex allergies in the population:

> *Studies show that roughly 6 percent of the general population and up to 15 percent of health care workers are allergic to latex, with the higher rate among medical personnel due to longer periods of contact with natural rubber.*

John Hopkins Hospital, Official Newsletter 22/01/08

However it is also interesting to note that latex can be found in various vaccines including Hepatitis B more frequently given to hospital staff.

Consequently, allergies are not so much an overreaction but a damage limitation reaction designed to stop these elements building up further within the blood, should we come in contact with them again, which could potentially cause more serious problems. One of the natural chemicals produced by the body involved in coordinating this response is histamine. However, orthodox practitioners often suppress these reactions using anti-histamines, for example. This disables the allergic response, the body is no longer able to react to these elements, and, unable to keep them out, they are given free access to the internal systems of the body. Again the sensitisation problem has not been solved but the symptoms are suppressed, the symptoms that were, as always, trying to help the body.

However, persistent suppression may lead to recurrences that may of themselves eventually prove harmful, for example as a result of suppression; the swelling from the inflammation could become excessive. Anaphylaxis is an extreme inflammatory reaction due to the extreme sensitisation of the individual, in such a condition airways could be blocked and then of course anti-inflammatories will suppress this reaction, which could save the life of that individual. However, note the ultimate dependence on drug intervention as a direct result of immune suppressive drug procedures in the first place. Drug dependency is a natural consequence of drug use, (i.e. suppression), the tendency to which, may of course be further complicated by nutritional deficiencies and inherited predispositions.

If the symptoms are successfully suppressed the illness is masked but the problem persists unrestrained. This could lead to a further internalisation of the problem, i.e. toxins that build within the blood system given access to internal organs and the nervous system; if you are fortunate, you may experience recurrent reactions, where the body tries again.

An accumulation of toxins beyond the blood and into the internal tissues of the body will be stored out of harm's way in the connective tissue, fat deposits and the joints. Toxins will also collect in the liver where the body attempts most of the detoxification reactions. Toxins and immune complexes will also collect by default in the kidneys where the fine capillaries filter out waste into the urine, and occasionally at the heart valves. Consequently these are the most common places where acute and chronic immune reactions occur. Here we see acute and chronic symptoms of cellulites, arthritis, nephritis, hepatitis and rheumatic heart disease.

The body has been doing its best to eliminate toxins, microbes and cellular debris from its interior thereby protecting the internal tissues of the body, and it is especially **important to protect** the cells of the **nervous system**.

When poisons, waste, cell debris and microbes build around the nerve cells, the failure of acute and chronic symptoms here could lead to neurological problems resulting in long-term damage, including paralysis, loss of sensory function, brain damage and even death. In the acute we see illnesses such as acute flaccid paralysis and infantile paralysis (*later called paralytic poliomyelitis in an attempt to attribute the pathology to the polio virus*), meningitis, encephalitis, and the chronic illnesses such as autism, attention deficiency syndromes, ME, Alzheimers and so on. These are the invasive illnesses that the body is doing its utmost to avoid, but in fact most suppressive medication, including vaccines, actually predisposes us to.

CHAPTER 16 - SUMMARY

➢ Vaccines were introduced when we understood very little about disease and even less about the immune system.

➢ Vaccines appear to have been successful because most of the reductions in illnesses happened as a result of increasing standards of living.

➢ The numbers of people contracting infectious illnesses are very small compared to those that don't, so it's not possible to gauge from direct experience whether vaccine benefits outweigh their side-effects, unless we look at the statistics.

➢ But vaccine reactions are under-reported, proper placebo trials are not carried out, safety tests are limited and conducted on healthy adults.

➢ Vaccine illnesses undergo reclassification which can create the impression that illnesses are on the decline.

➢ Vaccines can simply shift the nature of the germ associated with the disease, to a similar germ with a different name; so similar illnesses with different names become more prevalent.

➢ Vaccines contain known neurotoxins, poisons, antibiotics, preservatives, foreign gene fragments and other chemicals that can cause allergies, immune dysfunction, nervous system problems, brain damage, other illnesses and even death.

➢ Vaccines are injected past most of the immune system, therefore only stimulate a fraction of the immune system, and give the poisonous contents direct access to the internal organs and nervous system.

➢ Vital immune reactions to eliminate those toxins and learn from the procedure are unfortunately suppressed by pharmaceutical drugs because vaccine promoters do not understand immune function. They are obsessed with trying to stimulate antibodies, which is based on old immune theories.

➢ Essentially vaccines cause deeper problems that have historically been ignored by vaccine promoters because of the focus on short-term superficial goals.

CHAPTER SEVENTEEN

17 Why it's so important to be aware of your personal health paradigm

17.1 What is a paradigm?

Thomas Kuhn in his 1962 book the '*The Structure of Scientific Revolutions*' was largely responsible for giving the word paradigm its current meaning. The term refers to any general scientific and philosophical framework from which we study, interpret and understand our world. There are of course many different paradigms for a variety of world models, social, medical, physical etc. interestingly Thomas Kuhn believed that "Successive transition from one paradigm to another via revolution is the usual developmental pattern of mature science."

A change in paradigm was a radical shift in the way in which we perceived, understood and therefore interacted with the world, although the shift could appear dramatic, almost revolutionary, Thomas Kuhn and others have since realised that changing from one to another could equally occur in a more gradual fashion.

The germ theory, that diseases are caused primarily by the invasion of microbes and the perception of symptoms as being physical malfunctions during an illness, form part of the orthodox medical paradigm and therefore the basis of treatment; the administration of antimicrobial drugs to kill these microbes and pharmaceutical drugs to stop symptoms.

As we have developed technologies to investigate these phenomena, new paradigms emerge, and as is common to the emergence of new paradigms the old perspectives are not completely wrong but limited and therefore do not apply in ways that were previously thought.

17.2 Revisiting the assumptions of Pasteur/Jenner - Old and New Paradigm

Old Paradigm: The germ (microbe) is primarily responsible for infectious illness and can be transferred from one person to another. Therefore illness itself can be transferred from one person to another.

New Paradigm

> ➢ The accumulation of germs is the result of disease, but most live normally within the host, hence the dilemma faced in explaining 'carriers' of disease, clearly most of us have these microbes and have no symptoms of disease. We have reached a point where we are now vaccinating against common microbes that we have a normal tolerance of, for example the meningococcal and Hib vaccines. We also see that illnesses do not follow patterns relating to microbe evolution but directly follow disease conditions of the individual and their susceptibility patterns, therefore they proliferate where there is toxicity, emotional susceptibility, nutritional deficiency, immune suppression, immune failure and heredity.

In certain instances microbes can be ingested with decayed food along with their toxins, in addition normal microbes that inhabit the body can contaminate other parts of the body from injuries, all of these are special cases of microbial contamination (the microbe arriving with the material on which it lives). The so-called infectious illnesses such as measles, chicken pox, polio, tuberculosis, etc are entirely different to these, although the old infectious disease paradigm would like to treat them as though they were the same. Such microbes do not fly around the planet infecting individuals, indiscriminately causing disease.

Although microbes can be cultivated in someone with an illness and transferred from one person to another, there is no illness (even in epidemics) unless there is susceptibility and the illness expressed in the next person will be entirely related to their susceptibility. The range of possible symptoms varies according to the susceptibility of the patient.

Old Paradigm: Different microbes cause their own specific illness and therefore infectious illnesses are classified according to the microbe.

New Paradigm:

> ➢ Illness is inextricably linked to the patient's susceptibility, so for example; many microbes can proliferate in the digestive tract and the symptom response involves vomiting, diarrhoea etc, if the same toxins build in the blood the corresponding blood toxicity would be dealt with by forming a rash. If the same toxins and microbes become more invasive affecting the nervous system, symptoms of septicaemia and neuropathy may result. Consequently the conclusions of Pasteur are ultimately inaccurate in the more important details. Different microbes are associated with very similar illnesses (clinically indistinguishable) and the same microbe is associated with widely different illnesses in different people, an illness cannot be defined by the microbe alone.

Old Paradigm: Some microbes are more dangerous than others and can cause serious illnesses even in healthy individuals.

New Paradigm:

> ➢ Individuals succumb to illness in a manner that is based entirely on their unique susceptibility; the microbes present in the environment do not determine the severity of a disease. If

you are chronically ill with immune deficiency, then when in crisis, you will develop an acute illness and it will be the best response your body can manage and will be representative of the conditions you are in and your own immune capabilities. The response itself will not be the problem; the response could enable a step to increased health. Yes, the illness could also leave you in worse health, but that would be dependent on the conditions that provoked your response. The conditions are the problem not the response, suppress the response and you could make the situation worse. Getting a serious illness can only happen in seriously ill people or when exposed to severe and obvious trauma. In a seriously ill person, any number of toxins and even normal beneficial microbes could become invasive, causing serious illness, but this is entirely due to host susceptibility, (the state of health of the patient).

Drug companies use the worse case scenario to promote a vaccine or antimicrobial drug, creating the impression that the microbe itself is the element that determines how dangerous the disease is. This portrayal of illness feeds into our fear and if you look into where this concept is promoted you will nearly always find it is when selling medication, both pharmaceutical and natural. Sold on the line that "you never know when it can happen to you, even very healthy people can catch a serious illness". Although I have to agree you never know when 'it' can happen to you, you do know what kind of things can happen to you in terms of illness and under what circumstances. It is your susceptibility that determines how dangerous your condition is or will be.

Old Paradigm: New viruses not seen by the population before will have greater potential to cause mass epidemics and serious diseases because nobody would have developed any immunity to these novel microbes. This is because effective immunity requires that our bodies have been exposed to the virus before.

New Paradigm:

> Immunologists have demonstrated since the 1970's that the immune system of the body, knows what is foreign, because it works through a reference of self, anything that is not itself is foreign. The immune system constantly identifies foreign microbes even though it has never seen these microbes before, just as one would know someone to be from a foreign race even though they have never seen them before.

> The recent claims (2009) of the identification of a novel swine flu virus (contrary to predictions of the vaccine industry) resulted in mass infection, yet very low rates of disease and milder than normal severity of flu. We are in constant contact with all kinds of rapidly changing viruses without the concomitant manifestation of disease. The need to forewarn the body by injecting microbes and chemicals in the form of a vaccine is based on an outdated model of immune function.

Old Paradigm: The formation of antibodies to microbes is indicative of an effective immune response, therefore the detection and measurement of antibody levels is a measure of immunity within an individual.

New Paradigm:

> The large numbers of antibodies measured by immunologists seems to happen as a last resort in blood toxicity, microbes can be kept in appropriate places in the body without them ever having entered the blood and therefore without the need for antibodies. The general immune system develops from birth and with the increase in capability of immune function the numbers of toxins and microbes capable of entering the blood diminishes. Immunity is a learnt process that develops from childhood to adulthood, involving many more systems than just B cells and antibodies. Most people are immune to illnesses and have <u>no</u> associated antibodies.

The concept of presenting microbes (as immune challenges in the form of vaccines) to our blood, assumes that we need to see these microbes in our blood in order to recognise them and deal with them efficiently in the future and also assumes that we need to produce antibodies to every possible disease agent that we would like to be immune to, this is a completely flawed and outdated concept of immunity. Immunologists have demonstrated that the immune system learns from its immediate environment and learns itself, therefore is able to recognise non-self and does not need to see something before-hand to know that it is not required. Vaccines are based on an old theory of immunity that is in fact wrong. The more up to date concepts of immunity also acknowledges that immunity is a whole body response and can only be learnt, the learning is general and does not only apply to specific microbes. Therefore we do not need to suffer an illness to be immune and we certainly do not need microbes injected into our blood in order to learn immunity.

There is a new paradigm in health one that acknowledges firstly the interconnectedness of systems, the energetic and material, mind and body, and the vast ecosystem of our vitally important microbes as well as our own cells. If we want to understand immunity we need to understand how the body learns to deal with its environment, in order to understand that we can observe how we learn to do anything from learning to walk, talk and eat or any number of developmental issues. The new paradigm also acknowledges that the human body is intelligent and that symptoms are a coordinated attempt to deal with the environment, therefore in finding optimum health we need an optimum environment. Optimum health is the interplay of human activity in the greater ecology of the planet. Complementary and alternative treatments acknowledge why and how we are reacting as well as what we are reacting to, it is a more holistic, respectful, safe and effective method of treatment. This perspective opens many doors to people and creates possibilities in treatment that are simply closed without it. The difference in outcomes when adopting this new paradigm over a more simplistic treatment of the human being is as different as night and day.

CHAPTER 17 - SUMMARY

➢ The old germ theory of disease doesn't take into account the susceptibility of the patient.

➢ Germ theory mistakenly attributes the cause of disease to the mere presence of the germ; most people carry these germs and have no illness; therefore the individual has to be susceptible in order to contract the illness.

➢ Serious disease is a reflection of the serious nature of someone's susceptibility; you can transfer germs but not susceptibility.

➢ Many different germs can be associated with the same illness and one germ can cause many illnesses.

➢ Germs may have many different roles in illness; some may be beneficial, so attempting to eliminate them all, could be harmful.

➢ Antibodies are a small component of immune function, stimulating them artificially is based on an old immune theory that uses vaccines to mimic a crisis.

➢ The immune system learns through small challenges where crisis is neither desirable nor necessary; it is not necessary to get run-over in learning to cross the road.

➢ Symptoms of illness are often intelligent attempts of the body to resolve issues when pushed beyond normal limits. This has largely been unrecognised in a pharmaceutical approach to health care

➢ A certain amount of illness is an inevitable consequence in the development of a child to an adult, and the process of learning to deal with its environment, through 'trial & error' and 'trial & success'.

➢ Minimising the consequences of acute illness and reducing long-term chronic illness, is the goal rather than the total elimination of all illness - eliminating all error is inadvertently a futile attempt to eliminate learning.

➢ Attempting to eliminate all illness can lead to long-term problems - better a grief in your life than a life of grief.

CHAPTER EIGHTEEN

18 More New PARADIGMS in health care

"There is one thing stronger than all the armies in the world; and that is an idea whose time has come"

Nation 15 April 1943

18.1 Additional Strategies for treating disease and maintaining health

By incorporating up to date scientific discoveries of the human body and innovations from holistic medicine we can distinguish several facets of our new medical paradigm.

➤ **LOOKING AT CAUSES**
We live in a vast network of interconnectedness; all systems and therefore all cells of the body are connected to each other, microbes of the body are in intimate contact with our own cells, our internal environment of nutrition and toxicity is influenced by our external environment. Symptoms of illness and microbes in disease are reactions to both our internal and external environment, in order to understand disease we need to look at the ecology of our external environment and the ecosystem of human cells and microbes within our own body. It is important to understand how and why symptoms and microbes appear out of balance. When fish

are dying in the lakes we don't think of adding drugs to the lake we look to see what is in the environment that is causing disease.

➢ **SYMPTOMS ARE INTELLIGENT**

Symptoms of disease are also part of a coordinated and intelligent response of the body, designed to compensate for the stresses that we are subjected to and therefore symptom reactions are intended to keep you alive. Rather than suppress symptoms many holistic therapists now use techniques to help the symptom response.

➢ **CONNECTING MIND & BODY**

The physical, emotional and mental aspects of the body are intimately connected; doing something to one system necessarily affects another, the mind can help healing and can also create disease. Treatments and interventions need to assess their impact on all these systems and would benefit by utilising the power of the mind in healing, as well as understanding how the mind is part of the disease.

➢ **MATTER & ENERGY**

Physical matter and therefore your physical body, are affected by energy, can produce energy and is ultimately a manifestation of energy. Therefore energy from our environment, therapeutic equipment, remedies, food substances and energy that emanates from therapists can have beneficial affects on the body as well as detrimental. We need to be aware of how we can utilise energy, as well as physical matter, to aid healing and how to protect ourselves from its damaging effects.

➢ **GENES ARE NOT THE ULTIMATE CONTROLLERS**

Genes for disease can be expressed as healthy characteristics in appropriate conditions and healthy genes can express as disease characteristics in other conditions. The genes are a blueprint for your expression of life but not the ultimate controllers, they are influenced and changed by; environment, your responses to the environment, your perception of your environment and ultimately the activity of your mind. In your own lifetime you can acquire genetic characteristics of increased adaptability and improved health as well as acquire genetic characteristics of mal-adaptation and therefore poor health. These characteristics can also be passed on to the next generation and could have been inherited from the previous generation, finding a genetic basis for a disease will not give you the cause but an effect of previous causes. Changing disease characteristics can occur through changing the genetic expression without changing genes themselves, some conditions are easier to deal with than others; changing expression is much easier than changing genes.

18.2 What's alternative about alternative medicine?

The concept of suppression is one of the central themes of this book and the understanding of which is a prerequisite to the assessment of any medical treatment, orthodox or alternative.

The human body is capable of balancing its internal environment in response to any internal and external change; this balancing is part of its normal function and this self-regulation is called homeostasis. This ability to balance and redress disturbances continues into realms of greater disturbance, responding to more and more traumatic situations until the reactions are perceived as symptoms of disease, nevertheless they are reactions designed to bring us back into healthy equilibrium.

Through the symptom response, when equilibrium is reached, there is cure, and in acute scenarios we often accept that this can and frequently does occur. In more chronic and perhaps more serious conditions, cure unrelated to treatment is often described as 'spontaneous remission' and is frequently given no further significance.

Furthermore if patients are encouraged to heal by a placebo i.e. non-active medication, the effect although widely prevalent is naively considered to be an anomaly, as opposed to a reflection of the inherent curative nature of the human body. Instead it is used as an opportunity to research drugs that can out perform the placebo and rarely seen as an opportunity to learn how to enhance this self-healing response.

The human body is capable of 'self-healing' and as described in the earlier sections, this self-healing response is often mistakenly perceived as the problem, the suppression of which therefore leads to further problems. In orthodox medicine there is a tendency to think of symptoms as 'malfunctions' as though we are sophisticated machines and occasionally, through no fault of our own, things go wrong. However, we are beginning to appreciate the function of these symptoms and understand that these so-called malfunctions, for the most part, are essential reactions and therefore part of the cure. As such, humans, or any living creature for that matter, are **not** like machines, consciousness notwithstanding, i.e. we are not even just conscious machines, our bodies have the ability to adapt, learn and pass that information on to future generations.

The term 'Holistic Medicine' is significant here; it is used to describe the many therapies frequently called complementary or alternative and it is often thought that such practices are able to treat the whole person. In fact, all of our biological systems, however you care to define them, physical, mental, emotional and spiritual, are inextricably connected, therefore anything you do to one system will inevitably affect the other systems to a greater or lesser degree.

More importantly, the significant feature of holistic therapies is in the diagnosis of 'disease' and the assessment of treatment. In diagnosis, therapists assess as many of the influencing factors as possible, such as diet, toxicity, lifestyle, emotional state etc. and in their assessment of treatment, therapists consider the effects of treatment on the whole person over prolonged periods of time. Therefore by observing a more holistic (whole) picture, extending parameters and observing connections, therapists are able to see the many contributory factors and causes of disease whilst also being able to see the purpose and function of symptoms.

However, the pharmaceutical approach, addressing a single manifest symptom or collection of symptoms of one part of the whole, will miss the underlying causes and the purpose of each symptom. In addition, the effects of treatment will be narrowly confined to an expectation of its effect on that specific part of the body. Orthodox medical practitioners are therefore divided into collections of specialists as defined by physical divisions of the human body; skin specialist - dermatologist, kidney specialist-nephrologists, nerve specialist - neurologist etc. medication is then administered to affect either a physical, mental or emotional part.

But all pharmaceutical drugs have what are termed 'side-effects', the unwanted effects of these drugs. Because drug manufacturers only want a limited range of effects on a limiting range of symptoms, any effect other than what the drug company wants is called a 'side-effect'. The fact that all systems are related will however mean that the effects of drugs on one system will inevitably involve other systems and therefore will always produce other unwanted effects. More importantly the effect of suppressing a meaningful biological response could inevitably lead to the consequences of the failure of that response, the initial symptoms may go but others may replace it.

> *"The worst thing about medicine is that one kind makes another necessary."*
>
> **Elbert Hubbard**

For example, the function of the kidneys in cleansing the blood, is dependent on blood pressure; the greater the blood pressure the greater the filtration rate and therefore the greater the rate of cleansing. When blood toxicity levels rise and blood cleansing needs to be increased, kidney function can be increased by the production of certain hormones, (produced by the kidneys themselves), to increase blood pressure and therefore to increase filtration rate of the kidneys. Consequently some causes of blood pressure are a direct result of chronic blood toxicity and the resultant attempt of the kidneys to increase filtration. If the blood pressure is reduced with medication then it will be accompanied by increased blood toxicity that may give rise to an accumulation of toxins in the blood. This could then cause, for example, skin itching or even an accumulation of toxins stored in the joints giving rise to joint pain. These are in fact documented 'side-effects' of anti-hypertensives (high blood pressure medication). It may be a 'side-effect' as far as the drug company promotional literature is concerned but it is in fact the expected effect of the suppressive medication given the purpose of that symptom. This could even lead to the prescription of further medication to suppress these new side-effects.

18.3 Some principle differences between the orthodox and holistic

In naturopathic medicine the principle intervention is to aid function in disease, help elimination through the colon, or increase sweating, encourage foods and water to cleanse the body etc and as with nutritional medicine replace nutritional deficiencies. There may also be the need to adjust diet and lifestyle as these therapists acknowledge the connection between the symptom (i.e. the need for the reaction) and what the body is reacting to.

There are also situations where the body experiences difficulties reacting to physical, emotional and other immune challenges, due to blockages, with our energy tied up elsewhere in the body; acupuncture, shiatsu, etc. aim to enhance reactions by releasing obstructions to energy flow allowing the necessary immune reactions that are needed in other areas.

Physical tensions in the musculature can be reflective of mechanical stresses as well as directly relating to emotional and metabolic reactions, all of which can have a knock on effect on various organs. The work of physical therapists such as osteopaths, cranio-sacral therapists, and other energy therapists can release sufficient energy as well as relieve physical tension to allow the body to continue in its curative action.

Homeopaths will in fact administer a remedy that is designed to enhance your reaction so that, for example, a homeopathic remedy for some people with fever is belladonna, administering this will <u>enhance</u> the fever reaction, making it more effective. As a consequence the remedy speeds up the curative response and the fever (no longer needed) diminishes, in contrast to a pharmaceutical drug, such as paracetamol which is an antipyretic that will in fact suppress the fever response.

> *Reduce the fever – using aspirin, for instance - and the disease may last longer as Timothy Doran of John Hopkins University, Baltimore has demonstrated in the case of chickenpox.*
> **Journal of Paediatrics 114:1045-8 (1989)**

Indeed because there may be many different reasons for the body to produce a symptom, for example a fever could be part of the reaction to being chilled, an injury, food poisoning, toxins in the lungs, etc; they would actually require different types of fever remedies.

In addition, different individuals in response to the same challenge will react in different ways according to their own constitution and therefore will also require different remedies. Although there are similarities in patterns and responses, we are all unique individuals, with unique histories, unique constitutions and unique problems; a specific cure may work for one person but not the next.

18.4 An insight into homeopathy

It is worth noting here that homeopathy, from:

'Homeo' = *like, similar, same (Greek)*
'Pathy' or 'Pathos' = *suffering, feeling (Greek)*

Implies 'similar suffering' and is based on the principle often described as 'like curing like'. This means that a remedy capable of producing a pattern of symptoms in a healthy person, when administered to a person experiencing similar symptoms, will cure that person. Therefore the appropriate 'homeopathic' remedy for an individual is the remedy that is able to produce the very symptoms that patient is experiencing. The remedy therefore stimulates these symptoms even more, albeit quite subtly, i.e. the remedy actually <u>helps</u> your symptom response. This is of course in line with the intention of the healing body but, of course, diametrically opposed to most pharmaceutical interventions that do in fact suppress your symptom response.

As such, homeopathic remedies can be of any type, strength and concentration, and in fact other kinds of interventions can be homeopathic in principle, i.e. <u>helping</u> the symptom response of the patient. Some homeopathic remedies especially those of plant origin can be given in the concentrated forms known as mother tinctures and others are much more diluted, which has the effect of drastically reducing any possible aggravation of symptoms.

However, many more remedies are diluted to such a high degree that the original substance may no longer be present, this is often used as a justification for the assumption that homeopathy cannot work. Remember, however, unknown to many of the critics of homeopathy' the criticism of ultra high dilutions does not address the homeopathic principle but just these very dilute remedies.

If it is possible to continually dilute a substance until there is no original material left in solution and yet the solution still has an effect, this does appear to contradict all known chemical and physical laws. It is this issue that is continually raised by many orthodox scientists and doctors in a relentless, although unsuccessful, attack on homeopathy, yet homeopathy continues to gain in popularity around the world.

At first sight the continued dilution beyond the material presence would certainly appear to be irrational, however on closer inspection we can see that the phenomenon inherent in the dilution affect is pervasive throughout our world; it can be explained and demonstrated with present day chemistry and physics without negating what we already know in physics and chemistry. Just as it is possible to walk around a spherical earth and not fall off, without negating what would still happen if you were to walk off the edge of a cliff.

First of all we know these remedies have an effect on people and there are many controlled trials demonstrating their therapeutic effect in humans: Researchers from Limburg University Holland conducted a two year study and published their results in the BMJ 1991; 302: 316-23. They reported on 105 controlled clinical studies i.e. comparing to a placebo pill (a dummy pill) and found 81 showed that homeopathic remedies have a therapeutic effect beyond the impact of just placebo.

> *"The amount of positive evidence even among the best studies came as a surprise to us. Based on this evidence we would readily accept that homeopathy can be efficacious, if only the mechanism of action were more plausible. The evidence presented in this review would probably be sufficient for establishing homeopathy as a regular treatment for certain indications".*
>
> **Kleijnen J, Knipschild P, Ter Riet G.**
> **Clinical trials of homoeopathy**

However even these trials often fail to convince the sceptics and they believe that 'the placebo effect' is in fact the only way that these remedies can have any affect on a patient; so it appears many conventional practitioners have now conceded that homeopathic remedies can 'work', but it's through the belief of the patient and not the real affect of the remedy. However, clinical trials involving animals and babies also show effects beyond placebo, where the placebo effect, (i.e. due to the belief in the medicine in a baby or animal), would be minimal if not non-existent.

> *A study of homeopathically potentised remedies showed a reduction in the need for repetition of insemination and reduced semen loss in treatment of fertilisation of female pigs.*
>
> **Riaucourt A. L´Exemple de la Filière Porcine. Annals of the**
> **"Entretiens Internationaux de Monaco 2002", 5-6 October, 2002**

> *In a study of homeopathically potentised remedies the incidence of haematomas was reduced by 30 % in <u>turkeys</u> during transportation. The study was randomised, placebo controlled and double blinded.*
>
> **Filliat C. Particularité de l'utilisation de l'homéopathie en production avicole. Annals of the "Entretiens Internationaux de Monaco 2002", 5-6 October 2002.**

To further test the effect of the high dilution homeopathic remedies it is possible to conduct studies on cells in test-tubes, these are of course more objective effects, as they are not at all dependent on the belief system of a patient.

> *In a multi-centre study including four research centres in Europe the effect of high dilutions of histamine (10^{-30} – 10^{-38} M) were confirmed. Researchers were able to document that high dilutions of histamine inhibit human basophil degranulation. Results cannot be explained through molecular theories.*
>
> **Belon P, et al. FAC. Histamine dilutions modulate basophil activation. Inflamm. Research. 2004; 53: 181-188**

So there are of course plenty of scientific studies demonstrating the effect of the ultra high dilute homeopathic remedies; it would therefore appear that it is the lack of a physical or chemical model to explain the effect of the remedy that is the major stumbling block in its acceptance. However there are in fact experiments that are able to give possible mechanisms and quite easily explain the effect of the ultra high dilute homeopathic remedies.

For example, any substance with a repeatable structure can be studied with 'thermoluminescence', a method of heating previously irradiated substances which then gives off a pattern of emitted light that is characteristic of that substance. It is often used to study crystals and in an experiment involving ice with dissolved salts researchers in Switzerland found that the characteristic emissions of the salts lithium chloride and sodium chloride could be found even in ultra high dilutions when there was in fact no lithium or sodium chloride left in solution.

"As a working hypothesis, we believe that this phenomenon results from a marked structural change in the hydrogen bond network (of the solvent) initiated at the onset by the presence of the dissolved ions and maintained in the course of the dilution process, probably thanks to the successive vigorous mechanical stirrings."

Rey L. Thermoluminescence of ultra-high dilutions of lithium chloride and sodium chloride. Physica A 323 (2003) 67–74

As other experiments have shown, there appears to be an informational exchange that leaves an imprint in the water or other solvent, much the same way as somebody leaving an electromagnetic imprint of their voice on a tape or information on digital CD. You don't need to leave any substance you just need to rearrange the structure to impart the information; this can then have an effect on whatever is sensitive to reading that information. If you make a recording on tape, CD or even write a message in sand, you are rearranging the existing structure without leaving any new material, only those sensitive to the message can read it. A digital player can read a CD, a tape player read a magnetic tape and a human of appropriate literacy read the writings in sand. The action of homeopathic remedies is totally congruent to what we are now using in electromagnetic technology and informational technology of the 21st century.

Dr J Benveniste found that the therapeutic effect of homeopathic remedies could be erased by putting the remedies in a degaussing machine which is a powerful electromagnet used to erase magnetic tapes:

Water seems to be a kind of liquid magnetic tape using electromagnetic fields to store molecular information

The Federation of American Societies for Experimental Biology
1991, 5: A1583

Modern science is also acknowledging that the human body emits radiation and not just in a haphazard manner, consequently external radiation can resonate with this in ways that we are just beginning to research, the impact of specific patterns of external electromagnetic radiation are bound to be more significant when we realise that we are physiological bodies emitting and therefore sensitive to these kinds of energies.

> *This summer Dr Hyland will give two papers at international conferences outlining his research into the phenomenon that biological systems, including the human body, generate and emit extremely low intensity radiation in the form of photons (a microscopic packet of light energy), and that these photon emissions are not random but display coherence... the very weak emission of which can be viewed as an outward sign of an orderly functioning metabolism.*

Science Daily (Jul. 29, 1998)

The action of the homeopathic remedy also has an optimum effect at the correct dilution, this means that sometimes more dilute remedies have a greater effect than less dilute, because of the nature of less aggravation and the optimum frequency of the message. But it is also likely that continued dilution can have less of an effect than the previous dilution, therefore an optimum is required for the frequencies to match, this matching is called 'resonance', consequently it is not entirely true to say that, the more dilute the remedy, the more effect it will have.

> *"Living organisms are all a bit like radio receivers, and you can get resonance between external radiation and living things if the radiation matches natural frequencies,"*

Dr Hyland, Science Daily (Jul. 29, 1998)

The phenomenon of leaving an energetic or informational trace has also been demonstrated on the molecular level as well; in 1984 Dr. Peter P. Gariaev, PhD of the Russian Academy of Natural Sciences conducted experiments to show that DNA (the molecular components of our genetic code) is able to give off coherent electromagnetic waves that persists even when the DNA has been removed.

> *A quartz cuvette with a DNA sample is moved from one location to another. And a trace, a phantom, is left in the air in the original location of the sample. This phenomenon was registered using the laser spectroscopy method by P. Gariaev in 1984 in Russia and by the group of R. Pecora in 1990 in the U.S.A. Gariaev also investigated the stability of the phantom and he found the following. After blowing the phantom away by the gaseous nitrogen, it comes back in 5-8 minutes. And the phantom disappears completely after 1 month. We remark that sound waves radiated by the DNA molecules were registered in these experiments. (www.emergentmind.org)*

Further experiments have found that it is possible to transfer this information from one group of cells to another such that information enables healing or disease. Three series of experiments with identical protocols were conducted by P. Gariaev's groups Moscow, Russia (2000); in Toronto, Canada (2001); and in 2005 Nizhni Novgorod, Russia (2005).

> *A control group of rats was injected with a lethal dose of a poison called alloxan which destroys the pancreas, the organ responsible for insulin production in an organism. As a result, all the rats in the control group developed type 1 diabetes (high blood glucose concentration level) and died within 4-6 days. Then the same lethal dose of alloxan was injected to another group of rats. When the rats in this second group reached the critical condition, they were exposed to healing wave information. As a result of that exposure, the sick rats got healed: their blood sugar level got normalized and their pancreas got regenerated. This healing wave information was produced by a laser bio-computer when the laser beam scanned the healing matrix. The healing matrix was created when the bio-computer read information from the pancreas and spleen, which were surgically removed from healthy newborn*

rats of the same species as those used in the alloxan experiments.

Therefore as acknowledged by many scientists in this field, research demonstrates the electromagnetic and informational dimension of cells suggesting that cells do not only communicate by the movement of physical molecules from one cell to another or by nerve impulses but by coherent electromagnetic fields. This may be likened to the manner in which we are able to communicate with each other with radio, television and mobile phones.

Professor of Chemistry David Colquhoun in his criticism of homeopathy reflects the view of many in the pharmaceutical world and states in an article reported by Tony Edwards in WDDTY July 2006 "One of homeopathy's basic principles is the less you give of a drug the bigger effect it has. That's like saying the less whisky you drink the drunker you get"...

This is, of course, a misunderstanding of homeopathy and a confusion of two separate systems; firstly homeopathy is a therapeutic tool for enhancing the existing healing reaction of the body and can use concentrated tinctures as well as ultra dilute, the ultra dilution of remedies is not the homeopathic principle. Secondly the informational and energetic aspect of the homeopathic remedy needs to 'resonate' with an existing state in a patient to have any effect at all, the remedy is not just any old 'drug', an individual's homeopathic remedy only refers to an appropriate remedy that is able to elicit the same (or similar) symptom response that they are currently exhibiting.

In addition when there is similarity there is an optimum potency/dilution, which means that more dilute remedies can have a greater effect up to an optimum dilution, after which point, greater dilution can have less effect, therefore it is not a linear relationship of less is more.

We therefore need to recognise that information cannot be measured in weight and likewise material effects are not analogous to energetic or information effects. You can break a glass by dropping a heavy object on it or you can break a glass by directing sound waves at it, the sound waves that are similar to the natural frequency exhibited in the glass can break the glass. This is a well known, demonstrable, phenomenon that has been repeated and recorded many times. Sounds waves of greater frequency will not break the glass, neither will waves of less frequency, the sound waves have to be similar in frequency so they 'resonate' with the frequency of the glass, just like the necessity for the homeopathic remedy to stimulate symptoms similar to the symptom pattern of the patient.

Therefore even though sound waves and a heavy object can both break glass you cannot compare the two states in the same manner. Sound cannot be measured in units of weight and similarly it is not possible to have an optimum resonant weight of an object that can break the glass as you can have with the frequency of sound waves. What is true of weight is not true of sound waves and vice versa, because the more weight you drop on the glass the more likely it will break. The object breaks the glass because its force is proportional to its weight; this is not analogous to the resonant effect of waves.

Whisky makes you drunk because of its toxic material effect on the physiology of the body and this is not analogous to the effect of a homeopathic remedy, just as the information in a story can create feelings of sadness in a person which will have a measurable effect on the biochemistry of the body, you cannot measure the amount of story in 'weight of substance'. Nevertheless both physical substance and energy/information can and do affect the physiology of the body, the properties of them however need to be measured appropriately and likewise the properties of one do not negate the properties of the other.

The difference is in fact quite obvious, so there must of course be other reasons why elements of the existing pharmaceutical and medical profession choose to cling to an irrelevant argument to denounce the effects of homeopathy. The ultra dilute homeopathic remedy is easy to understand and does not in any way refute the physical laws of chemistry, just as the laws of electromagnetism do not refute the physical laws of the material world, but there are of course major implications in accepting the very real phenomenon of homeopathic and holistic medicine.

> If symptoms of illness are intelligent and beneficial, this would require we use medicines to work with the symptoms in illness as opposed to work against them and therefore most 'over-the-counter' pharmaceutical medications and many prescribed medicines could become redundant.
> If symptoms are reactions to our environment, it would become imperative to look at our environment and lifestyle, e.g. the toxic, emotional and nutritional influences on health; therefore most of the medical profession would have to re-train in their understanding of disease and use of therapeutics.
> If ultra dilute remedies have a therapeutic effect, medicines can be manufactured at incredibly low-cost, which would mean the pharmaceutical industry would cease to exist in its present format and could expect to lose vast sums of money.

The above is by no means exhaustive but is of course a significant incentive for many (although of course not all) in the existing medical profession to make sure that the public perceives homeopathy and similar therapies in the most unfavourable light as possible, thereby steadfastly keeping the debate in the banal arena of high dilution, desperately trying to convince the public that there's nothing in a homeopathic remedy.

It is of course as futile as trying to convince people that the manufacturers of their DVD have put nothing on it, which is actually true, there is no substance put on a DVD, you could conclude therefore that because there is nothing on it, it therefore cannot work. But like the homeopathic remedies the manufacturers would have rearranged the material, not unlike a message in sand, a message that your DVD player can read to give you hours of enjoyment, but they have most definitely put no 'thing' on it. So of course some ultra dilute homeopathic remedies may have no original substance but they likewise have a coherent energetic/informational imprint and as reputable experimentation shows they most certainly have an effect.

I have illustrated, albeit very briefly, some of the basic principles involved, in the therapeutic intervention of a few examples of complementary and alternative therapies, in particular homeopathy. All practises however recognise the importance of the 'symptom' as part of the curative response. The question as to how effective each therapy is, in the hands of which therapist, for what illnesses and under which circumstances, is beyond the scope of this book. However the important issue is to understand the principles in which they are practised and in turn understand the wider context of health and disease and therefore the basis of their success and increasing popularity.

Holistic therapists are able to see the connections between the various reactions of the different parts of the body, (disease symptoms) and what the body is reacting to (toxins, physical strain, mental pressure, emotional tension, nutritional deficiency etc), all systems are in fact integral parts of the whole, operating in a sophisticated and coordinated manner. Fever, malaise, lack of appetite, increased blood pressure, tightness in the chest, anxiety, may all be part of a synchronised response to a single event; however, we can only comprehend the function of symptoms in this manner when we are able to see the purpose of these symptoms as they relate to the whole organism.

18.5 In emergency

Orthodox medicine with its reliance on suppressive pharmaceutical medication appears to stand on its own when compared to the principles of almost every other holistic therapy. However at this point, it is worthwhile noting once again that this is not a wholesale condemnation of modern medicine. Firstly we are principally concerned with most over-the-counter and generally prescribed medicines, (the treatment of medical conditions) and vaccines (preventative medicine - prophylaxis), as distinct from laboratory and clinical diagnostic techniques, physical manipulations, nutritional, psychological and surgical interventions, in addition to accident and emergency medicine.

There are of course emergency situations that do require orthodox medical intervention, however, we need to make a distinction between 'accident & emergency' scenarios and medical emergencies as a result of illness. An increased likelihood of medical emergencies (as distinct from injury) is very often as a <u>direct result</u> of long-term drug suppression rather than due to the unavailability of this type of intervention, the lack of drugs is rarely the reason for the lack of health.

Referring back to our example of asthma and pharmaceutical drug use…

Asthma deaths are often thought to be due to under diagnosis, asthma we are told is a more dangerous condition than the public are aware of and deaths are due to insufficient medical treatment. However, post mortem investigations have revealed otherwise …the most common scenario being in individuals with a history of increasingly aggressive medical treatment rather than insufficient treatment.

Examination of their lungs after death revealed that their airways were plugged with mucus so thick and hard, that it could not be sucked up with the normal pipettes but had to be scraped out with a knife. This is in fact a direct consequence of drugs that are used to force open the lung tubes during asthma.

It is therefore not the side-effects of the drugs that are dangerous but the actual primary effect of the drug. The drug is working against the natural responses of the body, stopping the important tightening of the airways that enables the elimination of toxins and mucus during the coughing reflex.

In 1993 this lead Dr John Mansfield (President of the British Society of Allergy and Environmental Medicine) and Dr David Freed (Formerly lecturer in immunology, Manchester University) to come to the conclusion that:

"It is the doctors who have turned asthma into a killer. Any drug, that effectively reverses constriction and inflammation of the airways, renders the patient more susceptible to the direct toxic effects of the particles and chemicals that the inflammation was trying to remove, and therefore is likely to increase mortality".

Obviously there will be situations where the human body will not be able to respond successfully without medical intervention or where in fact the reaction itself is out of control, hence the appropriate use of orthodox medical intervention in accident & emergency situations. It is in this kind of disease management wherein the present medical establishment excels, however, they have expanded the application of this rationale to include all kinds of medical symptoms, treating every kind of symptom response as a mal-function that needs to be stopped.

However even in situations of severe physical trauma, understanding the concept of suppression and therefore the purpose of symptoms could also enhance treatment and could mean the difference between life and death. Professor Mervyn Singer, Professor of Intensive Care Medicine, University College London initiated a study in 2004 looking at the response of the human body in septicaemia (severe blood poisoning) with multiple organ failure. His scientists are looking back to the Battle of Waterloo, over 200 years ago, to investigate why their survival rates were so high.

> "Despite the non-existence of antibiotics, blood transfusions, life-support machines and other paraphernalia of modern intensive care, most of these soldiers recovered, often from life-threatening injuries...Yet with all our technical advances in medicine, mortality rates from conditions such as sepsis haven't improved dramatically over the last century"

There are many physiological reactions of the body to severe injury and poisoning; such as increased temperature, inflammation, immune responses, circulatory changes, hormone release etc and as Professor Singer agrees:

> "Even lowering the temperature in a feverish patient may be counter-productive"

What appears even more radical is the assessment of bodily functions during extreme shock, with lowered temperature, blood pressure and multiple organ failure, this is now being interpreted as an attempt to survive the critical trauma period minimising pain, blood loss and conserving energy. Professor Singer goes on to comment:

> "The remarkable thing about these organs that have 'failed' is that under the microscope they look normal and if the patient gets through this illness, the organs nearly always recover and return to normality so that patients aren't forever tied to a kidney machine or a ventilator, so there is a remarkable capacity of the body to recover"

> "Perhaps some of the interventions we're performing on our patients - be it mechanical ventilation, antibiotics, sedatives and so forth - are impairing the body's ability to adapt to a critical illness and so perhaps, in a covert fashion, **these drugs are compromising the body's ability to recover"**

If these reactions could be utilised instead of suppressed whilst also stemming blood loss and instigating surgical repair, survival would of course be <u>enhanced</u>.

Not only have pharmaceutical organisations used a medical emergency rationale to treat most other conditions and even misunderstood the purpose of symptoms in the medical emergency, but they are also expanding their drug market to include ordinary responses that should never be considered pathology, Ray Moynihan, a journalist, and Alan Cassels, a policy researcher in their book 'Selling Sickness' 2005 comment on this phenomenon:

> "The idea that drug companies help to create illnesses may sound strange to the rest of us but it is familiar to industry insiders. A recent Reuters Business Insights report designed for Drug Company executives argued that the ability to create new disease markets is bringing in billions in soaring drug sales. One of the chief selling strategies, said the report, is to change the way people think about common ailments and to make natural processes into medical conditions"

What may have started out as an over zealous application of a limited understanding of disease is being aggressively marketed today "to change the way people think" purely for financial gain.

CHAPTER 18 - SUMMARY

> There are in fact many new paradigms in health that have yet to make their way fully into orthodox medicine:

> Symptoms of disease are part of a coordinated and intelligent response of the body, designed to compensate for the stresses that we are subjected to and therefore symptom reactions are designed to keep you alive.

> Illnesses are a function of our environment as well as our unique susceptibilities; we need to look to our environment as well as the workings of our own cells to find underlying causes of illness.

> The physical, emotional and mental aspects of the body are intimately connected; doing something to one system necessarily affects another, the mind can help healing and can also create disease.

> Physical matter and therefore your physical body can produce energy, is affected by energy, and is ultimately a manifestation of energy. We need to be aware of how we can utilise energy, as well as physical matter, to aid healing and how to protect ourselves from its damaging effects.

> Genes are a blueprint for your expression of life but not the ultimate controllers, they are influenced and changed by; environment, your responses to the environment, your perception of your environment and ultimately the activity of your mind. Changing disease characteristics can occur through changing the genetic expression without changing genes themselves, some conditions are easier to deal with than others; changing expression is much easier than changing genes.

> Holistic therapies encourage the self-healing nature of the body through physical, energetic and/or psychological intervention. By observing a more holistic (whole) picture, extending parameters and observing connections, therapists are able to see the many contributory factors and causes of disease whilst also being able to see the purpose and function of symptoms.

CHAPTER NINETEEN

19 The Politics of Suppression – Who gains?

If we understand the purpose of the symptom response we are able to assess the ability of the body to overcome trauma and more accurately predict when it is failing, so that even in therapeutics there are situations where suppression may be desirable. For example, 'pain-killers' for certain conditions could actually enhance 'self-healing' in the short-term, if the cycle of pain and psychological stress are inhibiting healing, relaxation or sleep, fever suppressants may be useful in an individual with a heart condition, also the necessary medications in accident and emergency situations when the body needs support and supplementation.

However there is a vast amount of pharmaceutical drug intervention that is indiscriminately suppressive. This is often unnecessary and detrimental to health, as previously quoted, studies carried out between 1993 and 1998 reported in the Journal of the American Medical Association in 2000 estimate that deaths in the USA caused by side-effects of **correctly prescribed drugs** amounts to **106,000 deaths a year**. These are deaths that are directly correlated to the use of a particular drug and of course there are many more where the connections are not so readily seen.

Indeed a study reported on May 11, 2005 in the European Heart Journal (Vol.26, No.19 P. 2007-12) shows that **deaths due to sudden heart failure are three times more likely when taking prescribed medication for illnesses other than heart conditions**. These drugs are prescribed for nausea, vomiting, psychosis and for so-called infections. The study carried out in Holland equates to about 1,200 deaths per year when extrapolating to the UK.

And for patients that survive prescribed medication, pharmaceutical intervention may also lead to drug dependence, with an increasing likelihood of chronic disease and the need for surgical intervention. Much of this approach to health care is directly supported and intensely promoted by the pharmaceutical industry; we can see the logic in the well-worn rhetoric, the National Health Service is in fact a Disease Service.

Orthodox research will at best tell you what drug will suppress your symptoms better than a placebo; some drug research won't even tell you that; chemotherapy drugs for cancer are tested against other chemotherapy drugs for cancer, R Webster graduated twice from Brigham Young University, once in mathematics and once in accounting. He is the author of many physics and mathematics papers, and is the publisher of www.cancertutor.com He is well qualified in evaluating research and after extensive investigation of cancer literature he has come to the conclusion that:

> "***Never, never, never***, has a chemotherapy drug been approved by a study comparing the use of the drug on one group of patients, and comparing this group to a group of patients who refused treatments (in an FDA filing), nor has a study ever been done comparing chemotherapy to one of the top alternative cancer treatments (in an FDA filing)."

Is this fact known to doctors? To some yes…R Webster goes on to quote from cancer specialist Dr Glen Warner

> "We have a multi-billion dollar industry that is killing people, right and left, just for financial gain. Their idea of research is to see whether two doses of this poison are better than three doses of that poison."
>
> **Dr Glen Warner, M.D. oncologist (Cancer specialist)**

This research will not tell you what is, the best available treatment or cure and what the best life-style measures to adopt are. A disproportionate amount of time, energy and money is spent in trying to suppress responses with the justification of trying to avoid the worse case scenario, with virtually no effort in researching methods to create health and therefore truly avoid disease.

19.1 Politics of health care provision – domination of the health service by big Pharma

The health service as dominated by the pharmaceutical industry, is truly a disease service; it's main therapeutic function is to provide treatment that is suppressive and it is prescribed i.e. sold to patients, on the basis of what could happen in the worst case scenario, without providing options to increase health and therefore without providing options to reduce the likelihood of the worst case scenario.

In principle this kind of service will continue to increase in cost and these costs will rise faster than can ever be sustainable. If you take heroin to suppress the feelings you experience because of past and present trauma, unless the traumas are dealt with, you will continue to need more and more heroin until your health deteriorates to such a degree that more intervention and drug dependence ensues. Not to mention the financial inability to maintain the drug habit,

> *...our drug of choice may be different but the principle remains the same, as a tool to give us time, it may work, but as a principle of therapeutics it is doomed.*

In the five years, (2001 – 2006), the NHS drugs bill has risen by 46% to £8bn, it appears that if we were getting healthier we would in fact need less and less medication, why is the opposite the case? 'Reform' is an independent, non-party think tank whose mission is to set out a better way to deliver public services and economic prosperity, Henry de Zoete, is 'Reform's' Health Research Officer and has this to say about the demand for drugs.

"The demand for new drugs is insatiable, you only need to look at the Herceptin case at the moment to see that, but it is not sustainable."

19.2 Big Pharma Direct Marketing to the Public

The Herceptin story does in fact add another twist to the tale. The drug was hailed as a new wonder drug for breast cancer; it was different to standard chemotherapy. The drug attaches to receptors blocking their growth as opposed to just killing them. With some statistical manoeuvring, Roche, who had bought the international marketing rights, managed to turn apparently modest results into a wonder drug. However the real marketing tour de force was in utilising the sympathies of the general public, stories were leaked to the press creating such a public furore that eventually health authorities succumbed to the pressure and the drug was made available to the public paid for by the National Health Service.

The UK health authorities are guided by experts able to discern appropriate health care strategies, NICE.

The National Institute for Health and Clinical Excellence (NICE) is the independent organisation responsible for providing national guidance on the promotion of good health and the prevention and treatment of ill health, guidance is developed using the expertise of the NHS and the wider healthcare community including NHS staff, healthcare professionals, patients and carers, industry and the academic world.

Professor Peter Littlejohns, the Medical Director of Nice, published these comments in the Lancet Oncology 2006 7 22-3 and was initially opposed to its use.

"For every 100 patients prescribed trastuzumab [Herceptin], 94 will have been exposed to the side effects without any benefit, and at a cost of £400,000 per recurrence prevented."

In their seminar "Managing Scarcity in the NHS" on the 30th November 2005, Professor Littlejohns stated that the media were now a factor undermining their institution, because against his better judgment the NHS were to be providing Herceptin to patients at an annual cost of £100million.

Drug companies no longer targeted the experts, via support groups, charities and the press; they went straight to the public.

Expert analysis would <u>not</u> have given Herceptin the media hype and may never have granted the NHS license to supply this drug. The initial trials were neither blinded nor controlled, (as is common to cancer drug trials). Revisiting our earlier quote:

> "We have a multi-billion dollar industry that is killing people, right and left, just for financial gain. Their idea of research is to see whether two doses of this poison is better than three doses of that poison."
>
> **Dr Glen Warner, M.D. oncologist**

Herceptin was no different and in fact a closer look at the trials revealed that in addition to the lack of controls the trials were also very short lived and have been criticised because they were in fact stopped early. As reported in the Journal of the American Medical association (2005, 294: 2203-9)

> "These findings suggest clinicians should view the results of such trials with scepticism."

Tony Edwards of "What Doctors Don't Tell You" (August 2006, 17: 5; 6-9) reports on the hype, quoting Professor Smith Head of the Breast Cancer Unit at The Royal Marsden Hospital;

> "This is the biggest treatment development in breast cancer, in terms of the magnitude of its effect, for at least the last 25 years, perhaps as big as anything we've seen"

However Tony Edwards also publicises the only graph available showing the effect of Herceptin plus chemotherapy compared to chemotherapy alone. Remember Dr Glen Warner MD Oncologist

> ..."*Their idea of research is to see whether two doses of this poison are better than three doses of that poison.*"

After 10 months there appears to be the maximal difference in survival that quickly diminishes, and **after approximately 18 months just as many women have died that have taken Herceptin and chemo as compared to those only on chemo.** The results therefore show that under the trial conditions with no blinded controls, for certain types of breast cancer, 6% of people appeared to have survived a few months longer by taking a drug which has been inordinately hyped by the drugs industry and subjected to a huge placebo effect and at a huge financial cost with inevitable side-effects for most of its users.

With UK sales alone, Herceptin would have grossed £100 million every year and therefore made a considerable sum long before we've been able to see beyond the hype..."its effect...as big as anything we have seen", yet we have already quoted David Spiegel at The University School of Medicine, California 1989, who demonstrated that women with the **very late stage breast cancer <u>doubled survival rate</u>** when they took charge of their lives and used psychotherapy.

We then add this to the increasing use and cost in technology to screen for illnesses with the so-called hope of getting to the problem sooner. High tech screening may help in diagnosis but if allied to a therapeutic system based on suppressive medication, you are in fact only enhancing your ability to provide suppressive medication sooner. Screening does not screen for 'problems', screening looks for early signs of 'reactions' and therefore earlier opportunities to suppress which therefore creates more time to use more drugs.

Why does our health service operate in this manner? Most individuals within the Health service; doctors, nurses and the vast array of other staff, like any organisation are intelligent, well meaning and would like to contribute to the well being of their patients. However they operate under a consensus belief system, are constrained by health policy, dictated to by government, subjected to the pressures of a commercial world and more specifically pawns of a larger pharmaceutical industry.

In accident & emergency care, surgical procedures and bio-mechanical diagnostics down to the molecular level, modern medicine has a very useful role, but the application of pharmaceutical drugs to most medical conditions under the guise of a 'health service' is at best superficial. Orthodox medicine, under the guidance of the pharmaceutical industry, has devoted an immense amount of resources into finding out as much as possible about cellular reactions but with the objective of suppressing those reactions.

If the organisations that funded health research were interested in health they would find out about health, if they were interested in finding out about what psychological, environmental and nutritional factors affect our health they would soon make these discoveries. Clearly they are not interested in these issues, our health organisations, government health services, and pharmaceutical corporations have decided to keep research within the very small remit of cellular and physical symptoms, thereby defining a boundary between the human body and the outside world, such that, they at least, will make few connections between our environment and how we respond to it.

It is unfortunately of little interest to understand, pollution, insecticides, radiation, food quality, drinking water, emotions and the impact they have in relationship to disease. Our health services leave all of those issues out of the line of fire whilst concentrating on ever more technical and expensive means to suppress our responses, right down to the smallest biochemical level of our being. A question emerges; are there political, financial and other motivations that are keeping us firmly stuck in this status quo or are we victims of our own belief systems playing out the theatre of our slowly evolving consciousness?

19.3 Big Pharma Drives World Health Organisation (WHO) policy

In their drive for profit and market domination pharmaceutical companies have effectively hijacked the aims and objectives of doctors and health authorities. Many physicians and in fact government health authorities are, sadly, pawns in a billion dollar commercial industry.

Dr Marc Girard was commissioned as an expert medical witness by the French Judge residing over compensation claims for the families of those that died soon after receiving the Hepatitis B vaccine in France. This was the aftermath of a national Hepatitis B vaccine campaign conducted in September 1994 upon the recommendations of the World Health Organisation. The WHO, is supposedly a trusted and apparently autonomous organisation with the reputation of being impervious to commercial interests, its sole function is to research and implement policies designed to increase the health and reduce the disease rates of the world's populations.

Dr Marc Girard spent 1000's of hours on the subject with access to dozens of confidential documents, unfortunately what he found, in simple terms, was that the WHO had grossly overplayed the dangers of the actual disease and profoundly underplayed the dangers of the Hepatitis B vaccine. Dr Marc Girard had unearthed an efficient web of coercion exerted by the commercial manufacturers of the vaccine under the auspices of the WHO, in his letter to the Director General of the WHO he states.

> *"It is blatant that in the promotion of the hepatitis B vaccination, the WHO has never been more than a screen for an undue commercial promotion, in particular via the Viral Hepatitis Prevention Board (VHPB), created, sponsored and infiltrated by the manufacturers (Scrip n° 2288, p. 22). In Sept 1998, while the dreadful hazards of the campaign had been given media coverage in France, the VHPB met a panel of "experts", the reassuring conclusions of which were extensively announced as reflecting the WHO's position: yet some of the participants in*

this panel had no more "expertise" than that of being employees of the manufacturers, and the vested interests of the rest did not receive any attention."

Dr Marc Girard found further direct evidence of the ability of vaccine promoters to directly influence the WHO guidelines for their own profit in an interview published in a French Scientific Journal (Sciences et Avenir, Jan 1997: 27).

"Beecham's business manager claimed with outrageous cynicism "We started increasing the awareness of the European Experts of the World Health Organization (WHO) about Hepatitis B in 1988. From then to 1991, we financed epidemiological studies on the subject to create a scientific consensus about hepatitis being a major public health problem. We were successful because in 1991, WHO published new recommendations about hepatitis B vaccination".

Dr Girard therefore concludes:

It is sad news for people everywhere in the world that the WHO's experts needs manufacturers' salesmen to become aware of significant health problems. As a complementary check, you may be interested to learn that I was personally informed by the journalist responsible for this interview that the manufacturer did its best to prevent the publication of this stunning confession."

Surprisingly he discovered a similar deception in India reported in The Lancet 2004; 363: 659 by Dr Puliyel:

"In Feb 2004, I read a correspondence by an Indian colleague, Dr J. Puliyel (Lancet 2004; 363: 659), on the fallacies of the data spread by the WHO about the epidemiology of hepatitis B in his country. Although not well informed about the health situation in India, I was struck by the fact that the mechanisms of the deception as described by Dr Puliyel (gross

exaggerations, lack of references, inappropriate extrapolations), were exactly comparable to those I observed in my own country - and of course with the same results: a plea of "experts" to include hepatitis B vaccination in the national vaccination program, in spite of its cost and, I may add, of its unprecedented toxicity."

Further observations revealed that these were not isolated incidences, in his research Dr Girard was then able to see a parallel with another disease making the headlines at that time, 'avian flu' otherwise known as 'bird flu'.

It is quite easy to reconstruct that, under the lame pretext of increasing the manufacturing potential, the manufacturers managed to induce the WHO's experts to recommend flu vaccination, whereas it is plain that this immunization would have no protecting effect against avian flu.

In both situations, the trick was the same: to create a false alarm (about the inefficiency of targeted vaccination in the case of hepatitis B, about the necessity of increasing the manufacturing process in the case of avian flu), and to induce the WHO to plea for measures based upon misleading recommendations towards lay people (that everybody was at risk of hepatitis B in the former case and that flu vaccination could be useful in the case of avian flu)."

There are of course consequences to 'WHO' policy, their advice influences governments, and these governments, on the basis of this advice, set their own National Health Policies. Doctors and health personnel act on the guidance of that policy and they do so in the belief that the benefit of these vaccines outweighs their risk, they do not carry out further research and their advice to you the public is effectively the filtered down sales promotion from vaccine producers.

The aim of the vaccine producers is clearly to make more and more money; unfortunately this appears to take precedence over and above the recommendation of safe and effective health policy. Dr Marc Girard is not alone in his condemnation of the WHO.

> *"As a result, experts are currently challenging the WHO on the fact that deporting a veterinarian issue to a medical one prevented national agencies from taking appropriate measures concerning animals which, most probably, would have been far more efficient in limiting the spread of epidemics. In addition, it is sufficient to consider the figures of fatal reports following flu vaccination (Scrip n° 3101, p. 6) and to have a minimum of familiarity with the problem of under-reporting, to understand that up till now **irresponsible vaccination against flu has killed far more people than avian flu."***

Dr Marc Girard and Dr Puliyel are calling for an independent enquiry into the nature of WHO vaccine recommendations, in a letter to the Director General of the WHO, Dr Girard concludes:

> *"...the credibility of your organisation is highly dependent on an inquiry which differentiates between world health interests and those of WHO's experts."*

Many health care professionals are of course aware of the conflict of interests within a system of medicine that allows profit to dictate health policy. Some doctors themselves are distancing themselves from such practises and in fact a non-profit organisation has been established under the direction of Dr Bob Goodman, MD, a general internist practicing in New York City. His organisation operates under the banner 'No Free Lunch' (www.nofreelunch.org):

> *"Our members and supporters are physicians, pharmacists, dentists, nurse practitioners, physician assistants, medical ethicists, and others. Funding comes from membership fees, donations, and sales of our products. We receive no other outside funding".*

We believe that there is ample evidence in the literature contrary to the beliefs of most health care providers that drug companies, by means of samples, gifts, and food, exert significant influence on provider behaviour. There is also ample evidence in the literature that promotional materials and presentations are often biased and non-informative. We believe that health care professionals, precisely because they are professionals, should not allow themselves to be bought by the pharmaceutical industry: It is time to just say no to drug reps and their pens, pads, calendars, coffee mugs, and of course, lunch.

19.4 The Politics of Information Provision

Therefore many health care professionals are aware of the need to obtain unbiased information; however, it is quite apparent that the various health groups and commercial organisations have their own particular prejudices and preferences. Regarding our own individual health care choices we need to be able to understand the main issues and be able to ask the right questions. To date, there are no health authorities that provide services that are unbiased, with access to many different kinds of therapies, medicines and information on lifestyle. Therefore the responsibility to gain access to that kind of information is our own:

> **"As well consult a butcher on the value of vegetarianism as a doctor on the worth of vaccination."**

> **George Bernard Shaw**

> ➢ If you want to know about vaccines, speak to those that have an understanding of the research and are not subject to external pressure to produce or administer vaccines.
> ➢ If you want to know the standard government policy on vaccines, speak to doctors and health officials; they are all civil servants they work for the government and their knowledge is often little more than health authority rhetoric.

> ➤ If you want to find suppressive medication, talk to health care providers and pharmaceutical employees that provide those products.
> ➤ If you want to understand the consequences of suppression, speak to holistic practitioners trained in observing those effects.
> ➤ If you want to know about holistic medicine speak to holistic therapists.
> ➤ If you want to understand how lifestyle affects health, talk to those that work with themselves and others on health behaviour and lifestyle issues.

Our ability to understand the basic issues in health and disease will of course enhance our ability to make effective health choices, but currently that means collating evidence from other sources as well as from traditional medicine, because the National Health Services cannot provide that information on their own. By understanding the bigger picture we are enabled to search within a wider context and more easily find what is appropriate, safe and effective.

We live in circumstances where the existing medical establishment, both private and governmental, is intertwined with the corporate goals of the pharmaceutical industry, all of which exert a huge influence on the established media channels and therefore direct most of the messages that influence public opinion. For some the existence of such a pervasive bias could only be the result of an enormous conspiracy, but this is of course too simplistic, improbable and, on that basis, too easy to dismiss. The current medical paradigm is in fact an element of our individual and cultural development, one that is however rapidly changing. To appreciate the wider context of our medical predicament and the collective learning process, let us have a look at what drives some of our desires for the universal panacea and in so doing we shall be able to understand our current impasse and the direction towards a more positive picture of safety, increased health and abundant vitality.

CHAPTER 19 - SUMMARY

> The health service is now dominated by a huge industry set up around the orthodox paradigm.

> The medical industry, including the pharmaceutical companies, diagnostic and therapeutic machine manufacturers, health service staff, educational institutes, research publishers etc have become rooted in this paradigm, making it very difficult for them to adapt to developments in medical science.

> They have a responsibility to their public but also to their employees and shareholders which often pushes them to prioritise money over and above the incorporation of emerging facts elucidated by medical research, especially if those facts point to the necessity of operating in a different way.

> The extent of industry's influence on education, research, publications, media and government is often difficult for most people to comprehend. So members of the public, often unknowingly, are subjected to vast amounts of prejudiced information. This information influences their health care choices in ways that are often for the benefit of industry and not their health.

> There are obvious financial motivations for maintaining the status quo but equally important are the belief systems of most of those involved, belief systems embedded in an old paradigm that keeps medicine firmly in its orthodox track.

CHAPTER TWENTY

20 The emotional context of our personal journey to overcome disease

"When you trust in yourself you trust in the wisdom that created you"

Wayne Dyer

20.1 How we Lose Control of Our Own Health when we Invite in the Power Brokers of Health Care

During an acute disease emotional issues are in fact heightened; whilst suffering symptoms of illness we are apt to feel fearful, fear is in fact the single most important factor driving us to look for help outside of ourselves; fear of the symptoms persisting, fear of the pain getting worse, fear of deterioration, and ultimately, fear of death. However, fear is not an unfortunate artefact, confined to the cowardly or weak willed; fear is in fact an integral part of <u>all illness</u>, in <u>everyone.</u>

Unfortunately the emotional context of illness has been divorced from the process of healing just as fervently as the orthodox medical world has divorced the emotions from the understanding of the physical body. Pharmaceutical strategies for healing are therefore aimed at helping patients suppress symptoms and so avoid those feelings, and in fact exploit fears in order to coerce patients into a life of drug consumption; a pharmaceutical intervention adept at stopping reactions but unwittingly removing the possibility of resolving those fears.

We have looked at the consequences of acute disease and we know that it can lead to either;

> resolution and learning
> resolution but no learning
> unresolved chronic disease or
> death

In studying the patterns of illness we have been able to map acute and chronic disease and realise that illness starts in a certain manner and develops into deeper forms. We do not develop meningitis, autoimmune disease or cancer simply because we've not rested enough, eaten too much party food, or forgotten to wear our winter underwear, unless of course we already have a chronic susceptibility. Therefore homeopaths have observed and noted the patterns of illness that give rise to the first kinds of acute and chronic disease as well as many others further down the disease road. The symptoms of the first diseases have been observed and duly noted and these are called "Psoric" illnesses.

20.2 The Genesis of Disease

Psora is known as the root of all illness, original disease or original sin, from the unresolved issues of psora; all other illnesses follow, therefore, to resolve illness we are ultimately led back to a psoric condition and have to resolve the issues of psora. It is probably no coincidence that the bible story of 'original sin' parallels the observable symptom picture of the psoric illness. There are of course many interpretations of the story, and various accounts as to the truth of the story as compared to original messages from earlier writings, however there is nevertheless a useful message and without inferring any other religious connotations I would like us to look at the story of original sin and compare that to the observable symptom picture of psora.

It is told in the story, recounted in Genesis, the first book of the Old Testament, that Eve was tempted by a serpent to eat from the forbidden tree of knowledge. Tempted by the promise that she would become like god with access to knowledge hitherto unavailable to her, she promptly yielded to temptation and after a bite managed also to tempt Adam into the same act and accordingly to the same fate.

They immediately felt guilty and unworthy, embarrassed by their actions, unclean and ashamed of their very appearance they were compelled to cover themselves. Consequently they were cast out of the Garden of Eden by God and sent to wander in the wilderness, no longer in paradise, they felt alone, separate and abandoned by God. They journeyed aimlessly afraid of the unknown, afraid of the dark and fearful for their survival.

If we back-up in the story, we are also told that Adam and Eve were created in God's image and likeness and they were all knowing and they did of course have everything, the impact of temptation therefore hinges on one thing and that is "doubt" and more specifically "self-doubt". Once there is self-doubt the serpent was able to lead Adam and Eve away from their centre of self-knowledge, contentment and connection to God, which therefore instructs the human journey to self-realisation based on returning to the God-self in whatever guise that may be for you.

The observable symptoms of psora are mirrored by the details of the story of original sin:

- ➢ Self-doubt
- ➢ Fear of the unknown
- ➢ Fear of the dark
- ➢ Blame i.e. blaming others, (not taking responsibility), and/or blaming oneself, (guilt),
- ➢ Desire to hide oneself
- ➢ Appearance and/or sensation as if unclean
- ➢ Desire for food not satisfied by eating
- ➢ Hunger at night

➤ Fear will not recover from illness
➤ Fear of not having enough
➤ Dissatisfied, itch, desire for more

There are of course many more detailed symptoms; however the match is close and therefore significant. It is appears that the ultimate source of healing resides in the resolution of the initial symptom of self-doubt, finding confidence in oneself, knowing that you are able, that you will heal and that you have all that is required on your journey, the idea of acknowledging perfection in our being even though we have to grow and learn.

Even though an acorn is yet to become an oak tree, it is still perfect.

This theme is reflected, not only in our religious writings, but also in the origins of our supposed secular western culture. Dr Peter Kingsley is internationally recognized for his groundbreaking work on the origins of western spirituality, philosophy and culture. The recipient of many academic awards, he was a Fellow at the Warburg Institute in London and has been made an honorary Professor both at Simon Fraser University in Canada and at the University of New Mexico. He has worked together with many of the most prominent figures in the fields of classics and anthropology — speaking to Native American elders and physicists, professional scholars and followers of different spiritual traditions, healers and medical practitioners as well as people who very simply are aware of the need to wake up to a reality greater than the one we are used to.

Peter Kingsley in his book; "In the dark places of wisdom"…tells of the writings of Parmenides who pre-dates Socrates, Plato, Hippocrates and Aristotle, born over two thousand five hundred years ago in a Greek Colony of southern Italy, he is now famous as the founder of western rationalism—as the "father" of logic.

The teachings of Parmenides are significant in many ways; firstly they speak of innate human wisdom that leads us to knowledge of the self, the ability to heal oneself and access to increased human potential.

In order to heal Parmenides teaches that we need to 'incubate' our illness, meaning that we need to go alone, into the dark and touch the hand of Persephone (the goddess of death). Once again we see the requirement to resolve by being alone; healing is a personal internal journey that cannot be given to you by some thing or some one. 'To be in the dark' - so that we are able to see the light, the guidance from within. 'To touch the hand of the goddess of death' – i.e. to embrace the possibility of death, more specifically to embrace the consequences of error in our learning, allow the passing of the old and journey into the new.

There is only one courage

And that is the courage to go on dying to the past,

Not to collect it, not to accumulate it not to cling to it.

We all cling to the past

And because we cling to the past

We become unavailable to the present.

Bhagwan Shree Rajneesh

Kingsley finds that much of the wisdom passed on from our earlier teachers have been interpreted and misinterpreted according to our own limited belief systems and ulterior motives. The term 'incubate' has since been used as the period in which some external organism is busy creating disease within an individual before the symptoms of the disease are manifest. Persephone the goddess of death, which is the aspect of 'error' in learning through 'trial & error and trial & success', the doorway to new horizons, the ending of an era bringing in a new phase in our development, often misinterpreted as actual death being the healer...which of course it can be, but from the perspective of treating disease, not a useful criterion for healers.

Peter Kingsley, like others, advocates that in our search for truth and for ground-breaking discoveries, that we try to see our world with new eyes, rather than obsessively searching for new things in our old ways, only creating more details of the same limited story.

Self-doubt appears to be at the root of illness, consequently the resolution of which lies at the root of 'healing & self-empowerment', the South American Shamans (healers and spiritual guides) have a tradition that acknowledges a four step road to power, it is often said that knowledge is power but from the point of view of the shaman, knowledge is only the first of four steps to power. Knowledge is a pre-requisite to overcoming the first obstacle 'ignorance' but sufficient knowledge immediately presents you with the second obstacle 'fear', fear of not being good enough, fear that you will not cope, effectively what we have identified as self-doubt. The Shaman observes and consequently teaches that the only way to deal with the doubt is to 'take action'.

In all of our learning and growth we have recognised the trial & error and trial & success process that leads to self-development and therefore self-empowerment, the shamans have broken this process down and have recognised the essential component of fear, they have made the distinction between overcoming ignorance with knowledge and overcoming fear with action.

As we gain knowledge of health and disease issues, we are then faced with the need to act on that knowledge, but it is here that we are apt to feel afraid, it is at this point we often feel compelled to return to get more information and so begins the quest for ever more knowledge in the hope of finding the definitive piece of information that will solve our issue and hence resolve the fear.

However, after gaining the required knowledge, no further amount of knowledge can overcome fear; it is only resolved through action. Here we see the same message reiterated by Dr Susan Jeffers in her book "Feel the fear and do it anyway" here she states that the root of all fear is…'fear that you cannot cope', fear that you are not able, once again doubt in the ability of oneself. The trap, of course, is that we may convince ourselves that we lack sufficient knowledge and so we go back to look for more information, with more information we approach fear again, avoiding action once more we continue into a spiral of research, fear, the search for more information and more fear.

"Do the thing you fear and the death of fear is certain"

Ralph Emerson

Resolving the self-doubt, the fear that we cannot cope, is an integral part of our self development, consequently an integral part of our immediate symptoms of disease, and the degree to which it is unresolved, an integral part of our chronic disease. Avoiding fear in illness is the single most motivating factor that influences our desire for suppression, turning to experts other than ourselves, and this 'fear' often forms the very basis of our concept of disease itself.

The allopathic model of disease and its preoccupation with symptom suppression diverts the patient away from their process whilst increasing the underlying disease, motivated by fear of the process, the underlying fear increases. An all consuming endeavour to avoid a negative outcome with little or no energy in health creation, the outcome is predictable; avoidance of what we fear eventually takes us there. Understanding holism is one thing 'living it' is quite another.

The following example helps to illustrate some of these basic connections: If we imagine somebody that has no inherited or acquired chronic disease, they are in fact a rarity but are essentially pre-psoric; an emotional loss for example through a romantic break-up may cause them to comfort eat, over-eat sweet food etc. We know this can imbue a sense of comfort similar to the sweet breast-milk of mother, but may cause a build up of toxins in the blood, as sugar affects the acidity of the tissues, the functioning of white blood cells and the functioning of the liver (a main detoxifying organ) and could lead to a feeling of nausea.

> *"When a child is born his first love and his first food are the same thing – the mother. So there is a deep association between food and love."*
>
> **Osho**

Our person is afraid of being sick, of vomiting, and would do their best to hold down the contents of their digestion. This could lead to a mild blood poisoning and eventually an eliminatory rash with generalised inflammation, afraid of their condition the person could take an anti-inflammatory and even a drug to suppress the rash.

By treating the reactions as though they were the problem the patient could be successfully suppressed and could then acquire a state of psora. A chronic disease condition meaning that they are continually eliminating but at a very low level, therefore not efficiently absorbing nutrients, with continual low level inflammation and constant sense of not enough, low vital heat, fear of disease and fear of emotional loss.

Healing would require a gentle catharsis, eliminating the poisons which shifts the chronic functioning to acute which may then culminate in vomiting or diarrhoea, with the concomitant feeling of well-being and sense of empowerment and faith in their body's ability to heal. The underlying emotional loss may be more easily addressed with the increased self confidence and a realisation of the need to allow emotional closeness to others, resolving the fear of intimacy and the fear of disease.

This healing can occur through self-realisation by one-self or with the help of a suitable therapist; the journey is, however, very clearly a personal one and the learning can only occur by the individual concerned. Through suppression it is easy to see how unresolved disease can continue, along with the associated fears and insecurities, thus the fear that an individual experiences, in whatever path they are embarking upon, will be directly related to their history of resolved or unresolved issues, either from their own past or from their parents. Individuals will therefore experience more fear from the activities that resonate with their unresolved issues and so may feel a desire to avoid certain activities in their life more than others.

20.3 The Genesis of cure

We can see how self-doubt at a point of crisis can be recognised either as a pivotal point in our development and thereby allowed expression or exploited for the benefit of the apparent saviour. We can of course minimise the consequences of our error, reduce the steps such that error does not debilitate or kill, but once we are aware of the learning process we know that we cannot eliminate error without eliminating the learning process itself.

One cannot eliminate the error of falling over, in the process of learning to walk, only minimise the consequences of the error. Thereby in the development of the child to the adult, the child will be exposed to increasingly more environmental issues in their process from dependence to independent adult. There will inevitably be reactions that are indicative of trial & error and trial & success, the key is in reducing the steps to minimise the consequences of error, allow the reaction to resolve the error, and support the individual to gain self-confidence on the desired path to independence.

If we take for example a 'fear of the dark', we see that we do in fact have two choices; either use an external light or face the dark. Facing the dark will ultimately lead to the resolution of the fear and using the light will suppress the need to resolve it. By way of analogy we can see that we currently obtain our light from a utility company that sells us the energy for that facility, at a financial cost. These corporations could conceivably sell more of that utility and make more money by exploiting our fear of the dark; building on our self-doubt, compounding our internal story of inability and in so doing the power is literally handed over to a larger corporation because we perceive that we do not have the ability to resolve our internal issue.

But of course we could also use varying degrees of light to enable us to deal with increasingly darker environments, building the internal confidence to be able to face the dark, i.e. we would have learnt through trial & error and trial & success, using small steps. So the problem is not in using tools to help or to suppress, but in the intention and therefore in the overall goal of the intervention. To heal, one must understand the goal of self realisation and the ability of the body/mind to learn and heal, otherwise medical intervention is limited to the obsessive suppression of symptoms, often at a huge cost, not only a massive and ever increasing financial cost, but the cost of our physical, psychological and spiritual development with the inevitable deterioration in health.

20.4 Hindsight looking back at the Emotional Context of the Orthodox & Holistic Paradigms of Pasteur & Béchamp

"In all science, error precedes the truth, and it is better it should go first than last."

Hugh Walpole

In light of the emotional content of illness let us now look at the period of Béchamp and Pasteur and the germ theory of disease. Given that self doubt is such an integral part of the human condition, it is ever more apparent when confronted with our own symptoms of illness. Experiencing illness within the framework of Pasteur and Béchamp we are faced with two choices:

> ➤ Pasteur implores you to take a drug (poison) to kill the bug, you do not need to change any aspect of your life nor do you need to learn from the experience, the bug is the cause of the malfunction that you are now experiencing as symptoms of disease.

> ➤ Béchamp encourages you to adjust your external and internal milieu, that you can be responsible for your health and illness and the new paradigm invites you to trust that your symptoms are in fact healing reactions.

Even if you had an inkling that Béchamp could be right, you would still be faced with the doubt, "what if my actions do not work, what if I am not able to change, and what if my illness has nothing to do with me, what if it's just a dangerous microbe, what if the bug still gets me?"

The way of Pasteur was in fact the way of the disempowered and did in fact appeal to those not yet ready or able to see what resolutions were needed and those individuals that could see, but not yet ready to resolve, the core issues of their illness. On these foundations we have since created a dominant medical paradigm, one in which the body has been seen as an elaborate machine that occasionally, through no fault of our own goes wrong, with symptoms that are indicative of malfunction.

Drugs are seen as a positive way forward, with a cost versus benefit ratio that places the benefit of symptom removal against the cost of apparent, and under-reported, side-effects. A medical system established for the noble goal of palliation, relieving symptoms that are perceived to be unnecessary discomforts of the less fortunate, provided by practitioners professed to be more knowledgeable of our bodies than ourselves. Such an approach has inevitably led to the exploitation of unresolved fears, the disempowerment of the individual and could ultimately lead to the psychological regression of the mass medicated.

The mechanical paradigm dominant in medicine has yet to open its eyes to integrate the apparently disconnected physical and energetic systems of the human body to include the mental, emotional and spiritual aspect of the human being, one that is searching to learn and to be approved of. A physical body that operates in the same way as the mental, emotional and spiritual one, with a need to recognise the ability of the self and to overcome unresolved fears, through gentle processes of trial & error and trial & success, that necessarily leads to empowerment and increased freedom. As our societies have developed a technical and mechanical world view and superimposed that onto our medical system, these advances have created a void and a fatal flaw in our dealings with the human being.

CHAPTER 20 - SUMMARY

> ➢ Physical illness has an emotional component which is an integral part of the disease process; this element is often completely ignored by orthodoxy when dealing with the physicality of illness.

> ➢ Resolving the physical illness also involves facing up to the associated emotional challenges, the resolution of which helps to develop the emotional stability of the patient as well as the physical maturity of the body.

> ➢ Orthodox medicine attempts to deal with these emotions by either ignoring them or placing them in a separate clinical compartment where they are invariably suppressed with psychoactive drugs.

> ➢ Many other traditions, cultures and alternative practises are in agreement on the nature of this emotional context and the importance of resolving them in human development.

> ➢ But those in the medical industry often exploit the fear element in these emotions, in their attempt to mass medicate and control your symptoms. This is not an entirely mercenary process as those steeped in medical orthodoxy are on the one hand operating from the basis of their intense academic training as well as mirroring their own internal fears.

> ➢ The dominant medical paradigm is a product of a belief system that has overemphasised the mechanical reductive nature of the world. But, equally, it is a paradigm perpetuated by a medical profession who are themselves caught in the fear of disease. A medical orthodoxy dominated by individuals that have not yet integrated their own emotional development in the process of healing in their patients or themselves.

CHAPTER TWENTY ONE

21 The benefits of a shift to a Body Intelligence paradigm

> *"Men are not prisoners of fate, but prisoners of their own minds"*
>
> **Franklin D. Roosevelt**

21.1 Why modern medicine? - The emotional, cultural & spiritual context of our biomechanical world

The scientific bases for our technological successes have developed exponentially since the early days of Pasteur. Along with the advances in holistic medicine we are beginning to see how we can incorporate these linear mechanical concepts with the holistic and energetic qualities inherent in living processes and perhaps also see why we have been unable to do this so far.

We now understand that the systems of the human body are mechanically and energetically interconnected, that the psyche has much influence on our physical body, that matter itself is ultimately an expression of energy and that there are connections between particles that operate beyond the speed of light.

Physicists are in fact much more aware of the limitations of a mechanical model of the universe than proponents of orthodox medical practices, David Bohm quantum physicist and philosopher:

> *"Each part (of a machine) is formed (e.g. by stamping or casting) independently of the others, and interacts with the other parts only through some kind of external contact. By contrast, in a living organism, for example, each part grows in context of the whole, so that it does not exist independently, nor can it be said that it merely interacts with the others, without itself being essentially affected in this relationship.*
>
> *...Ultimately the entire universe (with all its 'particles', including those constituting human beings, their laboratories, observing instruments etc.) has to be understood as a single undivided whole, in which analysis into separately and independently existent parts has no fundamental status.*

Wholeness and the Implicate Order (2002) p.221 - David Bohm,

The approach to understanding our world from the perspective of breaking it down into smaller and smaller components is what we call 'reductionism', it will allow us to see certain mechanisms and from those insights develop mechanical technologies, bridges, engines, computers, etc. It is known to be a left-brained faculty and for many reasons, western society is predominantly left-brained in its approach; to understanding the world around us, to problem solving and social development. It has a more male-like quality when compared to the right brain which is more female-like, having the ability to see the wider perspective, find connections, and look at phenomena that operate over fields and distance.

> *"No, no, you're not thinking; you're just being logical."*

Niels Bohr

Many cultures have been excessively dominated by the male psyche and in our human development it has been argued that over the last 6,000 years there has been good reason for this; the 'perception' of scarce resources at certain times on the planet has been one factor leading to the formation of patriarchal, tribal groups that are able to accumulate food and commodities, defend themselves from the aggression of other groups whilst simultaneously feeling the need to aggressively dominate others.

The reductionist male psyche has dominated tribes, nations, corporations and similarly medicine. Likewise a pharmaceutically driven medicine disseminates a picture of the body that is mechanical and disconnected from its own systems; a human body that operates in fear of attack from external enemies and even in fear of attack from itself.

> *"We don't see things as they are; we see them as we are."*
>
> **Anaïs Nin**

By way of example, we know that many investigations since the publication of Pasteur's papers have shown Pasteur to have lied and faked his experiments;

- ➤ *'Pasteur Plagiarist Imposter'*, by R.B. Pearson

- ➤ *'Bechamp or Pasteur'* by E.D. Hume

- ➤ *'The Private Science of Louis Pasteur'* by Gerald Geison

> *"...I cannot but believe that the exposure I am making of Pasteur's ignorance and dishonesty will lead to a serious overhauling of all his work."*
>
> **Dr Leverson**

Yet these warnings appear to have been ignored and medicine has steadfastly followed a road that on the face of it has been demarcated by a Pasteurian paradigm. This was not the result of an all powerful conspiratorial oligarchy, but Pasteur played into the hands of a cultural belief system regardless of his honesty, accuracy or applicability. It is our mindset that has determined the nature of our medicine, interpreting microbes as foreign enemies that are intent on killing us, additionally a collective mind that perceives our symptoms as mal-functional system failures.

The paradigm taints our vision and colours our interpretations of the facts which of course influences much of our culture, not only in medicine. We can see parallels in agriculture, business, economics, management, politics, etc. For those of you in these various fields of interest you will see the analogies: 'Attack and defend' – 'them and us' – 'the enemy over there' – 'the problem existing out there'.

It is not a belief system that has no application, but a belief system with a very limited application.

However with such a mind set, medicine will be forever tied to hunting down biological opponents and apt to interpret the smallest of clues as positive evidence of the presence of a new adversary. So that even without direct evidence, it is inferred from indirect evidence. With for example the viral enemy, the establishment will not look at evidence to the contrary and inordinate amounts of resources are directed at finding solutions to what is interpreted as microbial attack.

Many cancers are now said to be caused by viruses, the new cervical cancer vaccine owned by Merck directed against human papilloma virus:

> Schoolgirls in Britain will be vaccinated against the virus that causes cervical cancer from September 2008, ministers have announced. This goes further than recommended by experts, with all aged 12-13 eligible, and a catch-up campaign up to 18.

A virus that even trained virologists admit, there is no evidence of, and is unlikely to be, the cause of cervical cancer:

> "...No set of viral genes is consistently present or expressed in human cervical cancers. S HPV does not replicate in the cancer cells...so the "hit-and-run" mechanism of viral carcinogenesis was proposed. It holds that neither the complete [virus], nor even a part of it, needs to be present in the tumor. Obviously, this is an unfalsifiable, but also an unprovable, hypothesis. All that has ever been shown is that HPV is sometimes present in cervical cancer tissue, but as we know it's also present in half the normal population."

Peter Deusberg PhD Berkely, University of California
The first scientist to isolate a cancer gene in 1970.
www.deusberg.com

With no microbial enemy they would of course still be looking for one; with the choice of having to address internal human issues or environmental ones the medical profession sponsored by the pharmaceutical industry would rather externalize the problem in the form of a single enemy for which we must find the magic bullet and there are a myriad different and creative ways of doing that. In principle the more one perceives from the point of view of 'them and us' and therefore 'destroy the enemy'; the more likely it will become a reality. If for example you perceive bacteria as the enemy and use antibiotics to kill them, we know that you ultimately disrupt your own bacterial ecosystem creating symptoms from fungus and other bacteria that do eventual become part of the problem.

It is of course out of balance with regard to the bigger, holistic, and one could say, more 'female' picture of the human being. By introducing a wider perspective and the recognition of the body's ability to intelligently and benevolently react and learn from its environment, we add meaning to the mechanical detail of human pathology. When observing whole body functions we are able to see the interconnectedness of our various physiological structures, we become aware of connections between body and psyche, the collaboration of our own cells and beneficial microbial systems, as well as an appreciation of the interdependence of the human being in its environment and other ecosystems.

21.2 Why we need a paradigm shift - The outmoded world view

Our current and dominant world view is responsible for many of the advantages of 21st century life but also creates perceptual shortcomings that are responsible for many of its failings. The dominant belief system is by and large mechanical, linear and simplistic; it underpins agriculture, food production, manufacturing, energy production, politics and many more facets of modern living. But it is also responsible for depleting resources without a strategy for sustainability; killing organisms without a concern for the impact on the larger ecosystem; dividing nations, life forms and the environment into them and us, thereby combating, poisoning and exploiting our world without considering the wider implications.

The Pachamama Alliance is a U.S. based not-for-profit organization looking at the destruction of the rainforests and recognise that it is driven by a complex web of social and economic forces, many of these forces are a logical result of modern society's worldview, a view that, although rich in technological insight, is often ignorant of the value of nature's apparently free and limitless services. They have created a symposium called "Awakening the Dreamer" that is also used by the organisation 'Be the Change' which helps individuals, organisations and cultures to make the changes critical to rebalancing some of the failings in many areas of modern life.

The description of the problems faced by many organisations also accurately reflect the problems with the dominant orthodox medical paradigm, the call for change and assessment of the problem moves away from conspiracy, malice and blame, towards a process of evolving from a fragmented and limited perception to a wider perspective whilst also incorporating technological advancement.

21.2.1 Awakening the Dreamer

It is as if we are living inside of a dream, sleepwalking toward oblivion, while self-serving, short-sighted interests encourage our slumber with managed news, celebrity culture and other weapons of mass distraction.

It has become clear that our political and commercial institutions are unable to effectively address this crisis, primarily because they don't realize that they are looking at an interconnected world through a fragmented lens. The villain here is not Big Business, the corporate media, the military-industrial complex, or even those who for personal profit seek to clear-cut our forests, overfish our oceans, pollute our atmosphere or drain our aquifers. The villain is an outmoded worldview - a way of seeing the world in which such unthinkable acts appear reasonable, sensible, and even intelligent.

Likewise a medical paradigm where injecting babies with mercury, aluminium, preservatives, foreign DNA, toxins and antigens; the suppression of intricately balanced immune responses; the killing of integral portions of your microbial ecosystem; the excision of important glands & tissues in your body, appears reasonable, sensible and even intelligent.

The awaken the dreamer symposium has developed out of a need to integrate the details of our technological way of life as well as the wider picture, recognising that all of creation is an interconnected web and each of us as an integral element in this miraculous and fragile weave of life. The parallels with the shortcomings of our orthodox medical world are striking, where there is a similar need to integrate the knowledge of microbes, molecules and symptoms of the human body with the wider perspectives of microbe ecology within the human body, the purpose of symptoms as they relate to intelligently keeping the body alive and the understanding of how all systems integrate within the human body and the wider environment.

21.3 The challenge to practitioners

The biochemical detail that we have learned from our technological world needs to be married to the 'meaning' gleaned from the wider perspectives of the holistic world. It is a necessary marriage of left and right brain, the domination of one over the other leaves us medically bankrupt and considerably diminished in our ability to heal and learn.

> *"Specialists (reductionists) are people who know more and more about less and less, eventually knowing <u>everything about nothing.</u>*
>
> *Panosophers (holists) on the other hand, know less and less about more and more, eventually knowing <u>nothing about everything.</u>"*
>
> **Paul Hague**

There needs to be a synthesis of the two, it is not simply a case of doing both at the same time; utilising reductionism and as a separate exercise bolting on holism or vice versa. In observing the purpose of physiological reactions in illness, the necessary path to resolution involves understanding the intelligence of the human reaction in illness.

If for example we understand the broader purpose of an inflammatory response, (with its redness, swelling, heat, pain and change of function) as well as its cellular biochemistry, we measure the success of our therapy in its ability to help that response to eliminate toxins, or to immobilise and heal injured tissue etc.

However, even as holistic therapists, if we take on the goals of orthodoxy, regardless of how 'natural' our remedies are, we become fixated on bringing down body temperature and reducing swelling. But this can occur **only** as a secondary result, once we have established healing. These results will **not** occur as a primary effect of our treatment **if** the underlying issue has yet to be resolved, unless you use powerfully suppressive drugs, but they of course will have consequences.

As such, therapists could, under the pressure of a medical paradigm, come to the false conclusion that their therapy is not working, if swelling and temperature are not immediately reduced, and therefore turn their patients over to the hands of orthodoxy with the patently more powerful suppressive drugs.

Within the criteria of the prevailing orthodox model the pharmaceutical profession will get to be right, alternative medicine does not work, which of course it doesn't, it doesn't work in suppressing the intelligent healing reactions of the human being.

Similarly if we understand persistent chronic reactions as a result of previously failed acute reactions and as an attempt of the body to minimise the effects of excessive trauma that we cannot yet resolve, we measure the success of our therapy in its ability to bring out and resolve underlying issues. If however we take on the goals of orthodoxy we are apt to direct our efforts at trying to stop these chronic reactions without a sense of the underlying issues, and will in fact attempt to prevent old reactions from resurfacing, which will again be in opposition to a natural healing reaction.

An alternative therapy in the hands of a therapist focussed on the aims of a pharmaceutically driven medical system will ultimately be unsuccessful in helping the human body and will ultimately fail. Therefore the challenge also facing holistic therapists is in understanding the detail of the pathology gleaned from modern science whilst incorporating a holistic perspective and knowing when to use which approach and when.

Alternative therapists are under increasing pressure to become regulated and standardised for the benefit of the public but also for the purpose of control. Those in positions of medical power would like to keep that control and will knowingly or otherwise enforce their own philosophy onto others. That philosophy will come in the form of teaching a standard pathology, teaching a standard diagnosis and consequently a standard rationale for treating disease, the alternative and orthodox will appear to come together, but of course they would not.

Medicine is in need of a paradigm shift towards the holistic, which is not a mere tinkering of medication, management or policy. When we understand the intelligence of the human body in disease, as well as health, it necessarily changes ones approach. This approach has been, and is still, of course, fiercely resisted and is why, for the most part, holistic medicine does not come from an alternative aspect of the medical establishment but from a new breed of therapist. It is indeed rare, although of course possible, to find someone that has been established in orthodoxy having made an equal transition to holistic therapy. Orthodox suppressive medication will ultimately find that its use is mainly confined to the emergency scenarios where in fact the body is failing. But even in such circumstances, emergency treatment of the future will also incorporate the holistic rationale that will account for the purpose of symptoms even in emergency situations.

We are challenged to understand the meaning of disease and therefore the path to health, we know this is not simply the suppression of the symptom. We need to know what the body is doing and why, thereby utilize techniques to support those reactions whilst reducing the presenting trauma and therefore increase awareness of what we are susceptible to, as well as addressing why. It is important to minimise the consequences of error whilst stimulating learning, which then enables us to overcome issues of susceptibility. We are in effect challenged to understand the 'detail' in the context of the 'bigger picture'.

The problems facing us medically and therefore developmentally as a human race, lay in the perspective of our patients' discomfort and disease, and ultimately in the perception of what we and our patients are humanly capable of. Physicians that use fear to coerce and control their patients do not understand the goal of health and the emotional context of illness, neither in their own selves nor in their patients. Health practitioners have a duty to empower and to help patients resolve the physical and emotional issues at the source of their illness, but in order to do that they need to understand the relationship of the psyche to the physical being, the ability of the body/mind to learn and heal, the consequences of suppression and therefore the consequences of exploiting fear in their patients.

21.4 The challenge to patients

Using illness as part of our development, learning to minimise reactions and reducing susceptibility to disease is a step by step process that can be learnt from issues of teething, walking, weaning, eating, schooling, working, nutrition, and so on. Unfortunately a pharmaceutically driven medical system exploits our fear of the reactions to these simple processes so that we are ultimately divorced from our innate healing and self-knowledge.

If we are **un**successful in our resolution of these issues we are unwittingly moved head-long into deeper and deeper crisis, until we feel no longer capable of trusting ourselves or the abilities or our children in illness. By the time we reach a hospital ward, we may feel it is already too late to embark upon a 'healing journey'.

Pasteur proclaimed to have the light to those fearful of the dark, the answer to those not ready to take on the responsibility for their health, whilst also providing a male hierarchical mechanism to disseminate power from many to the few, and since his time orthodox medicine has doggedly pursued the one and only linear path.

We need to judiciously use the tools of our technological world whilst also allowing us to resolve our own internal issues. As such we need to incorporate the teachings of the holistic with those of the reductive and therefore incorporate the view of Pasteur with the teachings of

Béchamp. The continued and inappropriate use of suppressive drugs occurs through our own ignorance, but once we have knowledge, they are used because of our own fear. Our dependence on a suppressive drug culture, pharmaceutical, street drug or otherwise, is a measure of our inability to see the meaning in our expression of discomfort and consequently an inability to resolve our own internal issues.

The trick to the development of self-awareness and self-empowerment, in ourselves and our children, is to learn and to give support through the minor shocks and disturbances of life, such that we move away from the possibility of severe medical crises. Then as we develop, physically mentally and emotionally, crisis becomes less likely and in the event of crisis, our ability to deal with it greatly enhanced.

It is with the simple issues that we, as patients, are able to learn about our health and healing, a process that is made much easier with the help of a suitable holistic health practitioner. Step by step, as we learn to deal with the small health challenges that we are faced with in our daily life, we experience the rebalancing process of disease and realise that our passage through the emotions of disease now leaves us without fear of disease. The resolution of disease endows us with independence, increased adaptability and a greater sense of self belief.

The use of holistic therapy in both children and adults may be far more significant and vastly more profound than the advantage of just a sweeter tasting pill.

The references in this book are an integral part of the subject matter, for this reason and also for ease of reading; all references are also written within the appropriate text throughout the content of the book.

Aaby, P. Pedersen, R. Knudsen, K. - *Paediatric Infectious Disease* (8:197-200) 1989

Bach, Jean Francois MD DSc - *New England Medical Journal* (347; 12) 19 September 2002 -

Barclay, AJ. Foster, A. Sommer, A. - *Vitamin A supplements and mortality related to measles: a randomized clinical trial. British Medical Journal* (294:294-296) 1987

Barsky, Arthur et al - *Nonspecific medication side effects and the nocebo phenomenon. Journal of the American Medical Association* (287: 5; 622-7) 6 Feb 2002

Belon P, et al. - *FAC. Histamine dilutions modulate basophil activation. Inflammation Research.* (53: 181-188) 2004

Bohm, David - *Wholeness and the Implicate Order* (2002)

Browning, Jeffrey L. – *B-cells move to centre stage. Nature Reviews Drug Discovery* (5: 564-576) July 2006

Chakravarti, V.S. Lingam, S. - *Annals of Tropical Paediatrics* (6: 293-294) 1986

Collier, Richard - *The Plague of the Spanish Lady*

Coutinho, Antonio - *European Molecular Biology Organisation Reports* (3:11; 1008–1011) Nov 2002

De Kruif, Paul - *Microbe Hunters*

Dole, Lionel - *The Blood Poisoners* (1965)

Doran, T.F. et al - *Acetaminophen: more harm than good for chickenpox? Journal of Paediatrics* (114:1045-8) 1989

Doyle, Patricia A. PhD. - *Tropical Agricultural Economics*

Edelman, K. et al - *European Journal of Paediatrics* (158: 12; 989-94) Dec 1999

Flöistrop, Helen et al - *Journal of Allergy & Clinical Immunology* (117: 1; 59-66) Jan 2006

Geison, Gerald - *The Private Science of Louis Pasteur* (1995)

Grata-Borkowska, U. et al – *Effects of Neuraminidase on Apoptosis. Journal of Physiology & Pharmacology* (58: 5; 253-262) 2007

Guarner, F. Malagelada, J.R. - *Gut Flora in Health and Disease. The Lancet* (360) 8 Feb 2003

Gupta, Ramyani et al - *British Medical Journal* (327: 1142-1143) 15 November 2003

Hamer, Dr Ryke - *German New Medicine*

Havinga, H. W. - *British Medical Journal* (314: 1692) 7 June 1997

Holt, EA et al - *Paediatrics* (85: 2; 188-94) Feb 1990

Hume, E. D. - *Béchamp or Pasteur? A Lost Chapter in the History of Biology*

Hunt, K.J. et al - *International Journal of Clinical Practice* (64: 11; 1496-1502) 11 April 2010

Hyland, Dr G. - *Science Daily* (29 July 1998)

Jeffers, Dr Susan - *Feel the fear and do it anyway*

Jefferson, Tom - *Influenza vaccination: policy versus evidence. British Medical Journal* (333: 912-915) 28 Oct 2006

Kingsley, Dr Peter - *In the dark places of wisdom*

Kleijnen, J. Knipschild, P. Ter Riet, G. - *Clinical trials of homoeopathy. British Medical Journal* (9: 302; 6772; 316-23) Feb 1991.

Kreger, Bernard E. Craven, Donald E. McCabe, William R. - *American Journal of Medicine* (68: 344-355) 1980

Kuhn, Thomas - *The Structure of Scientific Revolutions* (1962)

Lamb, Marion & Jablonka, Eva - *Epigenetic inheritance and Evolution: The Lamarckian Dimension* (1995)

Lewin, R. – *Shock of the Past for Modern Medicine. The New Scientist* - 23 Oct 1993

Lipton, Bruce - *The Biology of Belief*

Littlejohns, Professor P. - *Lancet Oncology* (7: 22-3) 2006

Lovelock, James and Margulis, Lynn – *Gaia 2*

Lysenko, E.S. et al - *Public Library of Science (PLoS) Pathogens* 22 July 2005

Macfarlane, John T. Lim, Wei Shen - *Bird Flu and Pandemic Flu. British Medical Journal* (331: 975–976) Oct 2005

Mendelsohn, Dr Robert - *The Medical Heretic*

Moynihan, Ray and Cassels, Alan - *Selling Sickness* (2005)

National Institutes of Health U.S.A. - *Autoimmune Diseases Coordinating Committee Report* March 2005

Nesse, R. - and Professor Williams, G. - *Darwinian Medicine*

NHS - *Public Health Network Newsletter* - 16 May 2002

Null, G. PhD, ND; Feldman, M. MD; Rasio, D. MD; Smith, D. PhD, Dean, C. - *Death by Medicine*

Odent, M. Culpin, E. Kimmel, T. - *Effect of immunisation status on asthma prevalence. Journal of the American Medical Association* (272: 8; 592-3) 1994

Odent, Michelle - *Primal Health*

Olshansky, S. Jay et al - *New England Journal of Medicine* (352: 11; 1138-1145) 17 March 2005

Padian, Nancy - *The American Journal of Epidemiology* (146: 4) 1997

Papadopulos-Eleopulos, Eleni - *Continuum* (Autumn 1997)

Pearson, R.B. - *Pasteur, Plagiarist, Imposter*

Pert, Candace - *Molecules of Emotion: The Science behind Mind-Body Medicine*

Rey, Louis - *Statistical mechanics and its applications. Physica A.* (323: 67–74) 2003

Robinson, Douglas S. M.R.C.P. et al. - *New England Journal of Medicine* (326: 298-304) 30 Jan 1992

Rønne, Tove – *Measles Virus Infection without Rash in Childhood in Related to Disease in Adult Life. The Lancet* (325: 8419; 1 – 5) 5 January 1985

Sears, M.R. - *Epidemiology of asthma. Recent Advances in Respiratory Medicine* (4: 1-11) 1986

Shaheen, S.O. - *The Lancet* (347: 9018; 1792 – 1796) 29 June 1996

Shelton, Herbert M. - *The Hygienic care of children*

Starfield B. - *Is US health really the best in the world? Journal of the American Medical Association* (284: 4; 483-5) 26 July 2000

Straus SM, et al - *Non-cardiac QTc-prolonging drugs and the risk of sudden cardiac death. European Heart Journal* (26: 19; 2007-12) 11 May 2005

UCB Institute of Allergy - *Allergic diseases as a public health problem. European Allergy White Paper.* 2004

Upton, Mark N. et al - *Intergenerational twenty year trends in the prevalence of asthma and hay fever in adults. British Medical Journal* (321: 88-92) 8 July 2000

Vovers, H. – *Wheezing, Sneezing and Cancer Risk – Still an Open Door. Journal of the National Cancer Institute* (91: 1916-18) 1999

West, Jim - *Images of Polio*

Lightning Source UK Ltd.
Milton Keynes UK
UKOW01f1516090916

282609UK00002B/240/P